The
HEALING
POWER *of*
Sound

DAVID & CHARLES

www.davidandcharles.com

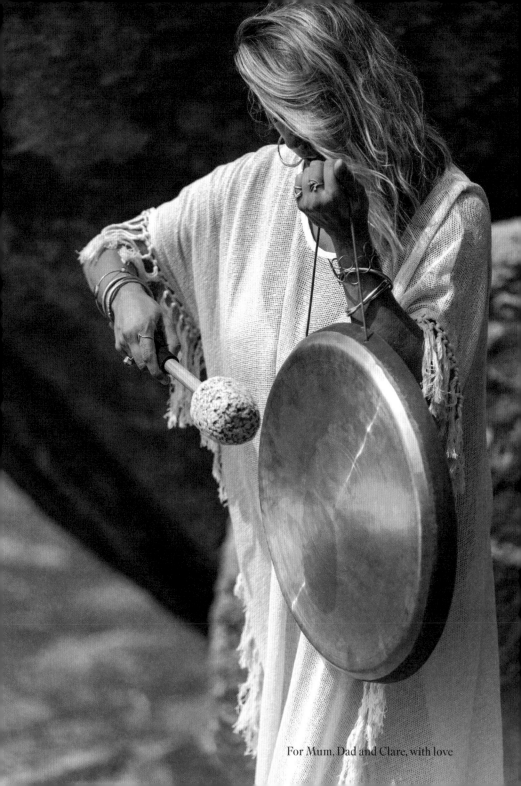

For Mum, Dad and Clare, with love

Contents

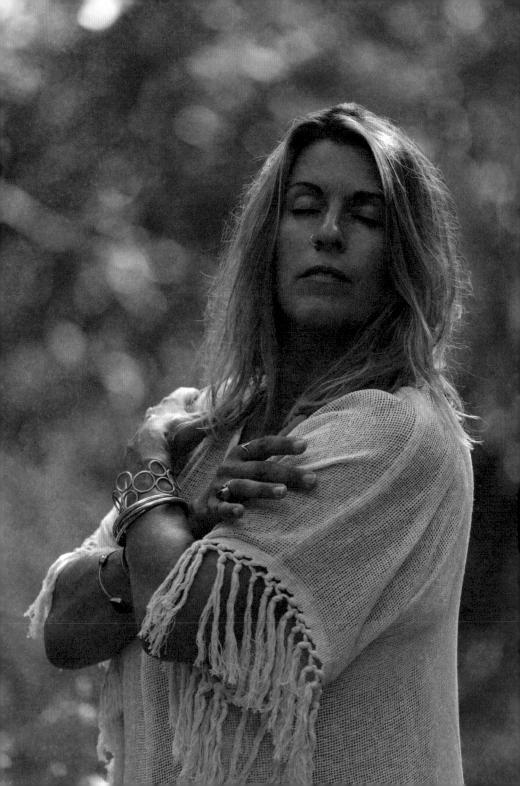

INTRODUCTION

Feeling Sound

" A person does not hear sound only through the ears; he hears sound through every pore of the body. " Hazrat Inayat Khan, sufi master and musicologist

Let's begin with a huge question. One of the biggest.

What's your favourite song?

I often begin my sound healing trainings by asking guests to share their response to this question, and it's always a wonderfully gleeful moment as I sense the room recoil in disbelief at the impossible task of choosing just one song from the myriad of melodies in their mind.

Can you do it? Just one song?

As we go on to explore sonic landscapes together in class, my students revisit this question from different perspectives, and by the end of the session it has become clear to everyone that the songs they are drawn to are simply a cipher for a deeper connection to an experience or emotion. The song is the key in the lock of their minds, the unique thumbprint that activates a specific memory or experience. It's a direct line to a relationship, place or feeling.

It's why selecting just one track from the jukebox of our memory is so challenging – we have a lifetime of memories across the full emotional spectrum from euphoria to bliss, agony and grief – each one connected to sound, music and potentially, a voice or lyric.

What I notice out of these sessions is that while so many people find it impossible to choose a single song, many find it really easy to name a sound from nature as something that captivates their attention and anchors their mood. It's probably not surprising that the most common sound my students identify as a favourite is the sound of the ocean, although the sound of birdsong at a certain time of day is also a popular choice. Usually with the scent of coffee and the texture of comfy loungewear woven through the memory too.

When we truly dive deep into the shadowlands of the mind, it's evident that sound is less about what we hear and more about how it makes us feel. Listening is a full body exercise that involves all of our senses.

This book is all about the incredible power of sound, and how we can understand and harness it for our own optimal healing. We'll explore the history, energetics and neuroscience of sound, and look at exactly how you can bring healing frequencies into your own life.

You don't need to be a musician, to read music, or even be able to hold a note to embark upon this journey.

You just need to be a curious human being.

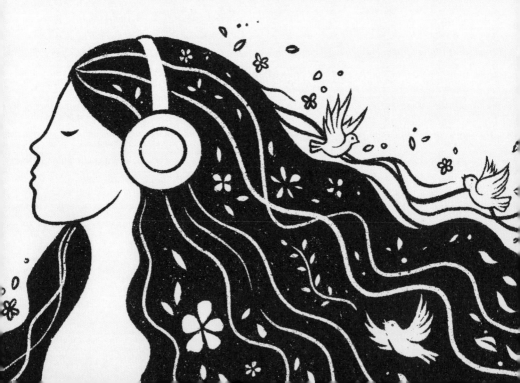

The Soundtrack of Your Life

Think about the sounds, songs or music that make you happy.

What happens when you re-play those sounds in your mind?
Does your body change? Perhaps you change position – do
you open or close your shoulders, heart, eyes?

Can you name the emotions or feelings that arise?

What happens when you bring the sound to life by
playing it on your speakers or headphones?

Invert the process: think about your happiest moments.
What sound, songs, or music do you attach to them?

If you can, try this for life's trickier moments too.

How does this make you feel now?

Don't forget to journal your discoveries.

We'll be stepping through lots of deeper exercises
around sound and memory later in the book.

Sound really is everywhere and everything – life itself is composed of sound waves.

Pause right where you are, right now, and LISTEN.

What can you hear? How does it make you feel? What emotion can you name, or perhaps just sense?

Even silence has a sound – some might say it's the most profound sound of all.

When we get deep into the cells that make up plants, people and places, we discover that they are simply oscillation, vibration, frequency; just a particle and a wave in a beautiful, eternal dance.

The world is sound – and so are you.

So what can you REALLY hear?

This basic science of frequency and vibration is exactly WHY human beings respond to sonic activity so profoundly. Sound has boundless power to alter our state of being, our moods, emotions and memories. As it dances through our cells it creates waves, patterns and movement that can make a simultaneously subtle and yet powerful impact on us at every level of being.

As we ARE sound, it is simply ourselves that we meet when we move with music, frequency and vibration. Attuned to certain sounds and frequencies, our minds open and our brains change gear – we are able to discover new extremities, layers and perspectives of being human. We can drop into the deepest states of rest and meditation, and the most illuminating aspects of consciousness.

This fluid, mutable nature makes sound a truly powerful medium through which we process our understanding of the world, and I don't just mean what we audibly hear through our 3D antennae (our ears)! Because sound is so much more than hearing – it's FEELING. We FEEL sound through the emotions that it stirs within us; through the effect it has on our own physiological harmony; and through the way sound can alter our brainwave states, fundamentally affecting our neural pathways and processes.

Sound is limitless (any attempt to measure it spins away into the mathematics of infinity) and yet it is also deliciously simple and accessible. Thanks to innate human connection to music, movement and voice, and the way we connect our experiences and emotions to the soundtrack of our lives, we can easily comprehend the natural mathematics of sound, making it a perfect tool for self-development, expansion and healing.

A Sonic Story

Working with sound to support health and happiness is something humans have known about since the earliest civilisations. People had sound long before we developed language, and ancient cultures have left us a rich tapestry of medicine, magic and intelligence that is steeped in sonic storytelling.

We know that wisdom traditions from across the planet worked with sound as a tool for healing, that temples and ancient sites often included resonant spaces apparently designed for certain sounds or harmonics, and that language, music and mathematics are innately intertwined with harmony and the architecture of the natural world.

Ancient civilisations from the first peoples of the Aborigine culture to the progressive healers of Ancient Egypt left us copious clues as to how sound was woven into healing practice at every layer of society. From didgeridoo dream-weaving to resonant water temples, Vedic vocal toning to transcendent Gregorian chants, sound was seen as a form of medicine. Traditional Chinese medicine has long understood the relationship between the five elements, five senses and beyond, and in the Chinese language the character for medicine is actually derived from the character for music, as Gao Yuan, conductor and composer with the Shen Yun Symphony Orchestra explains:

"Our ancestors believed that music had the power to harmonize the soul in a way that (traditional) medicine could not. In ancient China, one of the earliest uses of music was healing. The Chinese character for medicine actually comes from the charater for music."

Gao Yuan, conductor and composer

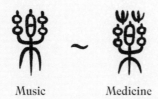

Music ~ Medicine

But over the passage of time, the rapid developmental pace of humanity has leaned into newer technologies and tools for healing, and in the race to embrace the future, modern medicine, the space age and AI, we seem to have collectively forgotten how to harness this immense and readily available natural resource.

For several centuries humans have marvelled at the progress of science and have defaulted to modern chemistry and an approach of cure over prevention when it comes to the wellbeing of both our inner soul and our external physical form. Don't get me wrong – we have created incredibly powerful medicines and capabilities when it comes to mending the human body. But it's my belief that just as all of nature's principles and laws are based around duality, the binary nature of creation – yin and yang, sun and moon, black and white – the healing space holds room for both East and West, ancient tradition and imagined future.

Here in the 21st century, we are finally beginning to remember the wisdom of sound. Amidst the wellness explosion of yoga, breathwork, tapping, gua sha and the rest, sound healing is having a zeitgeist moment, and is finally breaking through modern consciousness in a way that offers us so much fresh hope and opportunity.

From demonstrations on the sofas of morning televisions shows, to gongs and singing bowls soundtracking London Fashion Week, sound healing has never been more ready for its moment in the spotlight. It's becoming extremely easy to access high quality sound bath sessions from well-trained professionals, and it's so exciting that more and more people are being drawn into the powerful vortex of personal development and healing that sound frequencies offer us. But sound healing doesn't have to be something you can only experience in a yoga studio, or at a festival, or even in a therapeutic or clinical space.

Remember – you are sound, and sound is everywhere. It's everything.

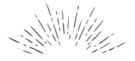

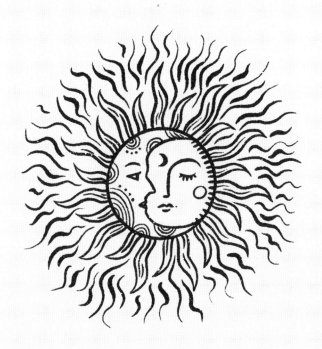

You can tap into your own sound healing journey any time you like. This book is intended as a guide, a workbook, to help you capture healing and harmony through a new connection to the sounds that shape your life, and a new awareness of the physical, mental and emotional impact that sound can have on your own personal experience of the world, and on your wellbeing.

To make best use of this book, you're invited to make it an interactive experience. Keep a journal to hand, and a set of headphones (good quality over-ear ones are usually suggested, but whatever you have is fine). If you have any instruments hanging around the house, dust them off and put them in your line of vision once again.

Most of all, cultivate curiosity, and awareness. Turn up your inner volume. Start to notice the sonic detail of your life.

What can you really hear?

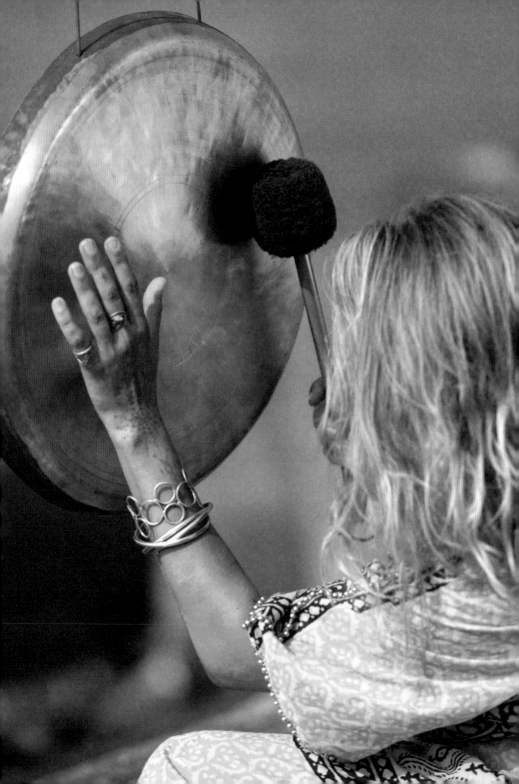

CHAPTER 1

The Science of Sound: 3000 Years of Listening

" Rhythm and harmony find their way into the inward places of the soul. " Plato, philosoper

Cast your mind back to your teenage days, and the dusty old science lab. I know – it wasn't my favourite place either, which is incredibly ironic! Do you remember the experiments with iron filings and magnets? Creating and directing current? Testing sound waves in a fish tank?

I never thought those long-ago days would be the fundamentals of my career and entire understanding of the universe, but then I certainly didn't realise what I now know to be the simplest of truths: THE WORLD IS SOUND.

Literally everything is sound, whether or not you can hear it. From the cells in our bodies, to the coffee cup in your hand and the tree outside your window. The universe is composed of boundless eternal dances between the particle and the wave; trillions of tiny interactions evolving from first meeting to relationship to endgame in the briefest of moments. Together the particle and the wave create an oscillation, a vibration that manifests as a sound.

The key to working with the healing power of sound starts with understanding what a sound actually IS, and while lots of spiritual and healing work may seem somewhat intangible and floaty, one of the most powerful things about sound healing is that it is underpinned by perfectly simple, beautiful science.

So let's start with what we know, which is that everything is a vibration, and has a frequency. You'll hear these words a lot as we journey through the sonic universe, so let's start by exploring the concept of what we mean when we say, hear or feel SOUND.

› Sound is... vibration travelling through matter

› Frequency is... the speed at which the vibrations travel

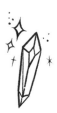

Pretty simple, right?

Vibrations are measured in hertz (Hz) and the hertz tell us how many vibrations per second are being transmitted by the sound (or the object transmitting it, to be a little more existential).

Let's bring this to life with the wonderful example of a Swiss watch – a beautiful piece of mechanical precision and artisan perfection. The watch runs on the oscillations of the tiniest piece of quartz – a powerful, almost microscopic fragment of nature in action (although as a disclaimer, lab-grown quartz is now more generally used in modern watches).

The quartz – the actual heart of the timekeeper – vibrates at a frequency of 32,768 oscillations per second – so fast it's imperceptible to the eye. In simple terms, it's that most subtle and yet potent vibration that runs the mechanism which in turn moves the second hand of the watch, literally putting time into motion.

The big takeaway is that the apparently static, miniscule crystal is in fact in constant vibration. When that vibration happens to fall within the range of human hearing (20-20,000Hz) it becomes something we can interpret with our built-in sonic antennae – our ears – and we call it SOUND.

However, ALL vibrations are sound. Humans simply don't get to experience them all audibly – but that doesn't mean we don't experience them in some other way! This is where the potency of sound healing begins to take root.

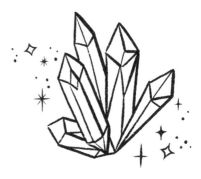

The Listening Experiment

› Look around your house with all your senses – walk around and explore room to room.

› What's making a sound?

› Write down the first five sounds you notice in your field of awareness.

› Now, sit still and close your eyes.

› Write down another five sounds you notice.

› Now tune into your own body.

› Write down what you can hear on the inside of your body (it may sound a little creepy or hard to get your head around – just trust, and give it a go).

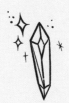

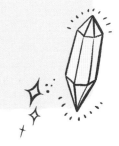

Here are my examples:

Initially, I notice the sound of kids in the playground next door to my house. I can hear the leaves of the trees in my garden rustling in the wind – like different instruments, the various trees and leaves have an array of notes and textures. I can hear birdsong and the less adorable sound of seagulls. I can hear the sound of cars, engines humming in the way of static queuing vehicles, rather than the roar of motion.

On my second pass, I notice the slight whirring of my laptop battery, although I think I feel it in my wrists as they rest on the trackpad, more than in my ears. Now I'm tuning in more carefully, I can hear the sea in the distance. I can hear the flicker of the flame in the candle that's burning on my desk – I realise that technically, I can hear the crackle of the wick.

Finally, I notice a rumble in my stomach. A little pop in my ankle when I go to move it – I haven't changed position for a while. There's a permanent rattle which I call white noise that's louder in my left ear than my right, kind of static, but low fi. I can sense vibration in my chest, and when I take a consciously deeper breath, I feel the sound of my lungs expanding before I hear the air on my lips. There's a slight tingle in my little fingers, but on careful study, my eyes tell me that they are definitely not moving.

Sound creates a powerful foundation for our lived experience, everywhere we look and listen there is vibration, information, being carried into us and through us. It's one of life's greatest open secrets that we don't just HEAR sound, we FEEL it.

In fact, neurologists indicate that our bodies were actually engineered to experience complex vibration rather than just straight-up auditory communication. Our ears capture sound waves, but their fundamental job is to process those soundwaves into electrical impulses that our brain can interpret. The sound that our brain tells us it can hear is almost like a coded cipher, one that defies language or translation – the sound itself is more like an external armoury, a spaceship that carries the secrets of emotional intelligence, memory, connection and communication all the way into the brain.

It's this decoding, deciphering, translation of sound into the brain's electrical intelligence that I think makes sound healing such an incredible tool. In the soundspace, we are not really listening to the sounds, but feeling them, experiencing them at an extra-sensory level.

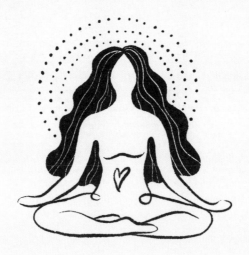

Before my sound journeys, new guests sometimes worry that the gongs may be too loud, or their hearing might be damaged during a session, as if they were down the front at a heavy metal gig in the 90s. I gently remind them that the sound is literally a perception – what we are really doing is sending very specific frequencies into the brain in a powerful code. Our brain is simply trained to tell us that the code has a sound, a note, a tone of voice. What might happen, when the brain stops supplying that feedback and context? What happens if we can experience the vibrations viscerally, physically, energetically, rather than through the messages of our mind?

This is something we'll revisit later on when we explore the role of the realms of consciousness in soundwork.

What's more, not all the sound codes we receive into our being arrive via the ears. With its voluminous water content, the human body is uniquely configured to receive sound through many routes – we are incredible sound conductors at a deeply cellular level, receiving vibrational messages on our skin, through our nervous and hormonal systems, and our wider sensory perception systems. Think about the way the hairs on your arm stand on end in a moment of synchronicity or emotional response, or the way you sometimes get a 'shiver' down your spine when you're not remotely cold.

Vibrations are messages, codes, wisdom and intelligence, frequencies landing on us and in us in every breath, every nanosecond. Our ears make it easy – but we would still feel sound and vibration without them. Just ask some of the many deaf and hearing-loss impacted musicians and sound healers out there. I'm one of them. The contemporary spiritual teacher Bab Ram Dass had this potent comment to make about the richness of silence, and I return to it often. See if it resonates with you:

"The quieter you become,
the more you can hear."

It's useful to land the point at this stage that sound moves incredibly differently in varying types of space, or media. The easy rule is that the closer together the molecules of a texture or material are, the faster the sound will transmit. Ever heard the phrase "I can feel it in my bones"? It's like an allusion to your inner-vision, or advanced auditory skills. Your bones may often feel a sound, sense a vibration, before your ears receive the tangible message.

While we're talking about the very bones of sound – the more dense objects are, the faster the vibrations are likely to be experienced, and this is why super hard structures like quartz and diamond are incredible sonic conductors. If you are into your crystals, this will make a whole world of sense as to why they transmit energy so effectively!

Sound has a slower frequency in water, and an even slower one in gases such as air, where molecules are substantially more distant from each other, and do not form physical matter beyond perhaps dust particles. As you reflect on your listening experiment, take a moment to consider the different types of matter in your own body – bone, muscle, blood, water, and yes, the air between organs, the air in your lungs and the highways (bronchial tubes) that connect them to source. Perhaps now you can start to appreciate how sound moves very differently through our physical form, and just why frequency can create such an impact on our human experience.

So returning to your own listening experiment – now you know that you can practice FEELING sound, give it a go. Experience sound. Listening is a full body process. Where does sound land in your body? Do you feel it first and then tangibly hear it, like a wave rolling in? Which sounds weave together to make up the tapestry of your life? Which sounds provide your permanent ambient soundtrack, and which are guest artists?

Listening with our bodies is a lost art form, one that the ancients knew all about. We'll explore what we can learn from their legacy as we begin to unfold the history of sound healing and how we can work with our body's incredible ability to process sound as part of our personal journey back to harmony.

"The highest goal of music is to connect one's soul to their Divine Nature."

Pythagoras, philosopher and polymath

Let's slink down the school hallway from physics to philosophy.

From the pillars of Mesopotamia to the Amazonian jungles, many of history's most important theologians and thought leaders shared an understanding of the presence of a profound vibration at the ground zero of the universe – let's call it the big bang, or perhaps the cosmic Om. I could write for days unravelling fascinating storytelling from a wondrous web of cultures from across Earth's timeline, but ultimately they all end up on the same landing pad: that is, whichever version of science or spirituality you subscribe to, there's little doubt that an energetic interaction, a dance between the particle and the wave, is somehow intrinsic to the universe bursting into being.

Some religions believe that the sacred sound was created by a deity, others that it was the primordial sound itself that created God. While we're not here to debate the beginning of life itself, the concept of some kind of vibratory sonic boom triggering the prismatic universe as we know it certainly has a significant place within thousands of years of study across classical physics, ancient theology, and more recently, quantum theory. A large majority of schools of thought from across the planet place vibration, sound and ENERGY right at the centre of the story of existence.

Let's take a supersonic journey through some key moments in our understanding of sound and music.

History's most lauded and oft-quoted philosophers from Aristotle to Pythgoras, Plato and Confucius had all observed the impact of sound and music on the human condition long before Newton and later Einstein had wrapped their equations around the possible relationship of sound to the space-time continuum.

Their collective lifetimes of insight and Instagrammable quotes could be pretty much summed up in a single statement: without doubt, music moves us.

Flashback once again to those teenage classrooms and you might just recall Pythagoras, or at least, his mathematical theorem. One of the first people on record to establish the connection between mathematics and music, Pythagoras' tuning became one of the philosopher's headline gifts to history, alongside his early astronomical ideas and the rather important fact that he was likely one of the first few folk to teach that the Earth was not flat.

The work of these philosophical creatives was critical in the understanding of sound and music to humanity. Early Greek philosophy taught not only that sound was far beyond just audible vibration – noise – but also that it had emotive, evocative qualities, as well as being part of a wider pattern of life that Pythagoras and his people could track and evidence in numerology, the planets and in nature. They were able to take threads of wisdom left behind by the likes of the ancient Egyptians, and begin to piece together a new science with its roots firmly in vibration, energetics, and their apparent connection to consciousness and the very core of existence.

Sound was therefore understood not as entertainment in the temples of ancient empires, but as a portal to growth, self-development, emotional freedom and healing, through the art and science of harmony.

Sound immersion was understood in the same way. People piling into stadium gigs, turning up their favourite track on their commute, or beating their PB in the rain on their morning run demonstrates daily – SOUND MOVES YOU. Not just physically, but emotionally, energetically, spiritually.

You've had those experiences too. Use the prompts on this page to explore them.

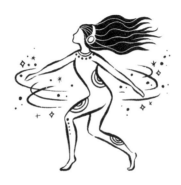

Explore Sonic Memory

Sit in a quiet place and take a few deep breaths. This
meditation and journaling practice is designed to connect
you to your emotions, through sonic memory.

Think about your favourite place. Close your eyes and
visualise yourself there now – it could be a beach, a café,
a room, with another person or people, or alone.

What can you hear? Organic sounds like plants, animals and weather.

What can you hear? Human sounds like voices, vehicles and activities.

What can you hear? Is there a song, or a piece of music, or a
single sound which embodies this place? Play it in your head
now. If possible, play it on your headphones or speakers.
Recreate the experience of being present in your place.

How do you feel? Can you name your emotions?

Now turn the music or sound OFF – literally and
in your head. What has changed?

Freewrite for a minute or two, keep your pen on the page and
explore what arises. If your mind wanders, put your sounds
back on and plug yourself back into your place.

"The Force is not a power you have... It's the energy between all things, a tension, a balance, that binds the universe together."

Luke Skywalker in *Star Wars VIII: The Last Jedi*

Brace yourselves: it's the science part. Unexpectedly but beautifully, the opaque field of quantum physics (which we are about to demystify) actually has a huge amount in common with some of the earliest recorded philosophical teachings, as well as much eastern philosophy from the Vedic and Chinese traditions.

It was at the turn of the century, in the decades around 1900, when physicists began to intently study the nature of matter, taking what had previously been an objective study of physicality into unchartered territory. Instead of exploring the natural world, space and time in terms of tangible, measurable physical form, these trailblazers forged a theoretical approach that was all about possibility. Seeing was no longer believing, and with Einstein's theories transforming the physicist into a global rock star in the early part of the 20th century, a new world order was born.

Thus was created the field of quantum physics, a disorienting and incredible area of subatomic science and mind-bending multiple realities. It sounds intimidating, even to me! But I've always used the helpful filters of cinema to soothe the overwhelming scale of this particular corner of science.

Just cast your mind through Superman's connection to the planet Krypton, Star Trek's light beam transporters, and the energetics of the Marvel universe. I've always especially enjoyed Dr Strange's energy-wielding symbols, which seem to me an alternative vision of reiki or runes. Within these accessible cultural references you can easily find examples of a broad universal energy that we are all beholden to.

Of course, the ultimate reference is the eternally vague and yet utterly captivating 'Force' that dominates all nine chapters of the greatest saga on chaotic family dynamics that cinema has ever seen. A mesmeric battle of yin and yang, light and dark, particle and wave, Star Wars provides an endlessly useful tool for comprehending the concept of interconnection across the galaxy, in all directions of space and time.

You're probably wondering – how did we end up HERE? Star Wars, Einstein and universal energy?

It's simple really. From Plato and Pythagoras to Nobel prize-winning particle physicists via the eastern philosophy of the Vedas, the secrets of the pyramids and Luke Skywalker, humanity has always had the sense that we are at one with the universe, that there is no space between ourselves, the stars and each other, that we are eternally connected by an invisible force. What modern science has shown us is that the force itself is a particle and wave – a vibration: SOUND.

What's more, we now know that these subatomic particles are in conversation. That once connected to each other, they are inextricably linked, as we all are, in a boundless tapestry of time and space, woven together through sound.

With the foundations in place, it's time to embrace this uniquely euphoric blend of science and spirituality and jump aboard the magic carpet ride of sound healing.

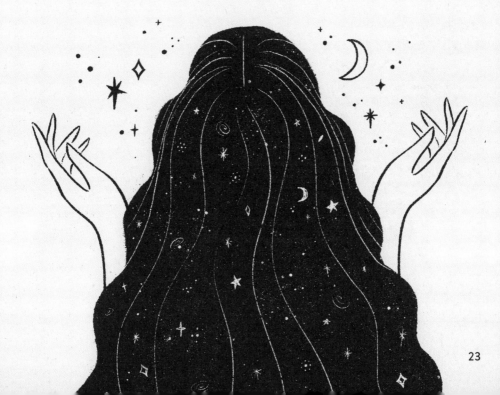

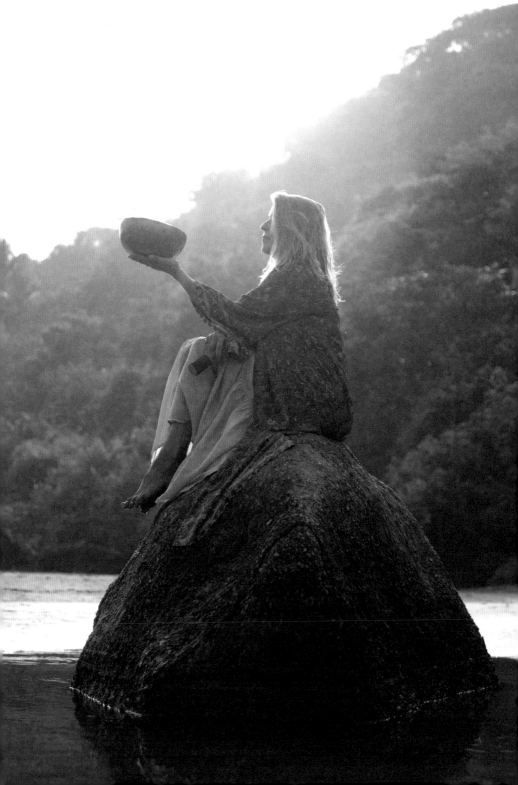

CHAPTER 2

Science, Meet Spirit

"One reason sound heals on a physical level is because it so deeply touches and transforms us on the emotional and spiritual planes."

Dr Mitchell Gaynor, oncologist and author

Let's be really clear.

Sound HEALING is one thing. Sound THERAPY is another.

They are non-identical twins, with polarised personalities and different haircuts. They both have their place in the wellbeing record box but they are not utilised in the same way, or for the same situations. They speak of two sides of the same album – science and spirit, the ancient and the future, the analogue and the digital.

In most regards the easy way to put some air between healing and therapy is to use the warp-speed progress of music technology as a cipher: you could say that sound healing is like the vinyl, cassette and ghetto-blaster generation of music. Sound therapy is the mp3, the digital synth, the iPod.

Or is it the other way round?

Sound healing has a very spiritual, cosmic quality about its process, which sits predominantly in the realms of supra-consciousness and transcendence; while sound therapy is grounded in science, clinical benefits, the mathematics of time and the electric nature of the human body.

Sound healing and sound therapy manage to be completely different, and yet co-exist in glorious stereo harmony, ultimately BOTH offering significant contributions to our potential for self-development and living a more gloriously WELL life. A potted definition of each follows, to help you get really clear on the range of soundwork out there for your exploration and wellbeing.

SOUND HEALING SITS AT THE INTERSECTION OF SCIENCE AND SPIRITUALITY

Science offers us such an incredible wealth of tangible, well-evidenced tools to support our personal development on this planet via sound; while spirituality, or what you might call energetics, provides alternative channels that take us beyond the limitations presented when we process the world solely through our five functional senses.

It's as if they are two adjacent rooms at a club – one playing old school house bangers, the other delivering a B-side of spacey arthouse grooves. Equally enticing – yet not exactly easy to move to simultaneously.

Part of my personal manifesto as a professional sound practitioner has long been that I work at the intersection of science and spirit, which is exactly where I think modern wellness is best located.

In this perfectly pitched place between practical pragmatism and the boundless vision of the quantum physicists we met in chapter one, we can reach for inspiration and information from both the material world and the realms that lie beyond the current edges of human experience.

So taking it back to the dance floor at our wellbeing club, I'm pretty sure there's room for science and spirituality to coexist on the decks – the perfect sound for the disco of the future, mixed by the ultimate DJ: sound healing.

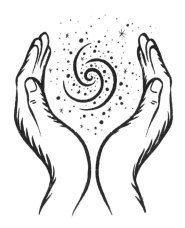

The Difference Between Healing and Therapy

> SOUND HEALING is where a facilitator creates an immersive soundspace – a sonic environment where, unplugged from the constant noise of the five senses, the recipient is able to move into their natural vibratory balance as well as into a harmonious subconscious state. This means that the recipient's physical and energetic systems shift into an optimal condition for self-healing – because a harmonised body can execute its own cellular function better than a stressed body. Thus in this highly supported state, a series of apparently cosmic physical, emotional and energetic shifts can take place incredibly quickly.

> Sound healing is often delivered in group sessions which you may see described as sound baths, gong baths or sound meditations, and the defining feature of a sound healing session is the potential for more transcendent, meditative or spiritual experience. You could also include binaural beats or sounds from nature in the wider sound healing bracket.

> SOUND THERAPY is better suited to a 1:1 experience, where the facilitator or practitioner works directly on the body and in the personal biofield of the recipient, creating targeted vibrations on specific areas of the body with instruments such as smaller singing bowls or tuning forks. These create vibrations, ripples at specific physical sites, amping up the experiential impact in addition to the wider harmonising one described above.

> Some practitioners may combine sound therapy with energetic work such as reiki or may use acupressure or marma points to deliver the vibrations consistent with ayurvedic or Chinese medicine teachings. Others may work in a more biomechanical manner, applying vibration topically at the site of conditions or physical concerns, or combining it with massage or chiropractic style manipulation.

> You could also define group work for specific conditions such as dementia or Parkinson's disease as therapeutic AS WELL as healing work, as it sits across the two aspects of sound, offering therapeutic outcomes via healing methodology.

> Additionally, there is a growing hybrid space that I'm referring to here as VIBRO-ACOUSTIC THERAPY, which is where frequencies are delivered to the body using beds, chairs, blankets, cushions or even on-body wearable devices which are digitally programmed with frequency cycles designed to regulate the electric fields in the body. This exciting field of vibro-acoustics sits closer to the therapeutic side of sound, as it does not usually involve a transcendent experience and is derived from clinical settings, where much of the research into this work has taken place.

> As a practitioner of both healing AND therapeutic modalities, this is my personal take, and reflects how I help people to get clear on what sound can do to support their individual needs. You may find other variations or interpretations, and I encourage you to stay curious and open-minded as to your OWN opinion and the way in which you bring sound work into your life.

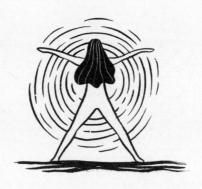

Let's address one of the main challenges that 21st century wellbeing is always shadowboxing with: HEALING. This we might define as the process of fixing or making something better. Tangled up with the notion that perceived spiritual or energetic practices like sound, are in some way an intangible, hyper-real bandage that we are all too susceptible to.

HEALING is a pretty omnipresent word isn't it? Perhaps even a slightly muddy, if not downright dirty one.

From a social media standpoint that's awash with healing-focused accounts and brands, it does often feel like EVERYONE is talking about healing from something or other, that we are drowning in a navel-gazing, introspective culture obsessed with labelling its own condition as some kind of unique melancholy that demands a free pass.

You might know this as 'spiritual bypassing', and it does rather make the business of speaking about work like sound healing that little bit tougher!

The explosion of wellness, casual colloquialism around eastern spirituality, and the slow seeping of ancient practices into the new millennium seems to have created something of a healing epidemic, as much as it has offered a solution to one. From the planet's rainforests and oceans to our capitalist culture, decolonisation, gender politics, mental health and ancestral wounds – everyone and everything seems to be crying out for healing in some shape or form, and it's certainly difficult to spend any time online without tripping over a healing hashtag or the latest embodied leader offering a six-figure solution to your spiritual malaise.

Regardless of sound's scientific basis, healing certainly has 21st century buzzword status and when it comes to introducing myself as a sound healer I have to swallow the ick factor in a big way. The word HEALER implies that I'm here to fix you, to actively do the work for you, but I've never seen it in those transactional terms. What I really love about sound is that in the space, you become your own healer, discovering that the medicine you need is within your own body, vibrating in your own cells, firing through your own consciousness.

The practice of sound healing is remembering your own harmony, returning to your own natural orchestration. Together we dance with your inherent energetics and frequency, until you arrive at a place where your body is vibrating in such a way that your physical, emotional and energetic functions are maximised.

MIC DROP: the sound healer's role is not to heal you, but to provide you with the optimal conditions for SELF-healing.

As your sound healer – or as I prefer to say, sound healing practitioner – I'm just here to steer, guide and support you by giving your bodily vessel its power back, selecting instruments and sounds with intention and precision and weaving them together to curate an attuned space in which you can return to your own homeostasis. Here, your cells, your organs, your lymph, your nervous system, can all serve their purpose more efficiently, without the constant prickle of external distraction.

So next time you hear someone call themselves a healer, get your guard up and check in to see whether they are offering a silver bullet, or a tool for empowerment. Because sound healing really is the latter. It's YOU in the driving seat, and your intention is the key in the ignition.

Of course, you can tap directly into sonic healing power all by yourself too, through making conscious decisions about sound, music and the spaces you inhabit in the wider landscape of your life. We'll be exploring what you can do to create your own self-healing spaces and practices deeper into the book.

For now, it's a great time to get your headphones on and tune into what it is YOU'RE here to heal. As we'll discover, intention is everything when it comes to working with sound healing, so find yourself a track that feels inspiring, brings you bliss, a big smile and ideally a drop of calm, and commit a few notes to your journal.

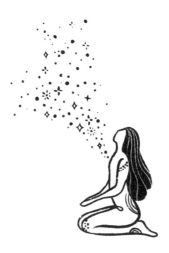

Crafting Intentions

Intentions are an incredibly important part of participating in sound healing. As we'll discover, so much of what happens in the sound journey exists in the liminal spaces beyond our conscious mind, so the seeds we plant there are fundamental as we invite the sounds to carry us into lucid dreamstate and beyond. Use these prompts to explore your intentions for your next sound session:

1. What are you calling in or manifesting?

2. What are you letting go, or preparing to release?

3. How would you like to feel on the other side of your sound journey?

4. What guidance are you ready to receive?

5. What does your heart want to know?

Back to the classroom for some social context on why we NEED sound healing, and your practical shortcut tools to start tuning in.

This dive into social history is a recap on the natural physical, emotional and energetic states that we have forgotten, how we've got there, and what sound healing can return us to. Let's get into it.

We already know that sound is everywhere, and that plenty of objectively smart folk through the last few centuries of human history thought it was a pretty tidy tool for wellbeing. But then we got distracted – by building cities, civilisations and computers; by fighting over money and power and figuring out how to have more of everything, and faster.

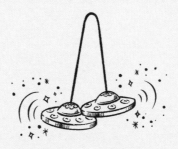

Somewhere in the last few hundred years, humanity put sound down and got into calculators. When we re-emerged, blinking into 21st century society, a LOT had gone down in the mists of progress. In the broadest of strokes, it seemed as if fear had held a mass takeover. A collective aversion to the unknown or the intangible seemed to have manifested, and the profoundly modern tumbleweed of ANXIETY had made its case for dominance, becoming not just an emotional response but presenting in our bodies as ill health and malfunction.

At least in the developed world, we had become reliant on pharmaceuticals, machines, and by someone with more letters after their name than us telling us about our own internal condition. In increasingly large swathes of the world (let's stick with calling it the developed world), people stopped trusting in nature, in the resonant wisdom of our ancestors, in the absolutely reliable rhythms of nature.

How did we get here?

Perhaps that doesn't really matter. What's important to note is that evolution has simply brought us to a generation of technological overwhelm. Too much of everything, and an endless hustle culture that has yanked us unceremoniously out of our natural state of being. We weren't born this way.

In fact, we were born with our own unique harmony, our own vibration and inner orchestration, a frequency as unique as our fingerprint or the iris of our eye. But – and I'm writing in generalised terms to help illustrate the state in which we find ourselves – our parents, peers and programming have all had an impact on that beautiful bespoke tuning. As we have moved through life, our tone has changed, maybe even our fundamental note. We've shifted collectively and individually from melodious rhythm to some kind of heavy metal space opera.

Fortunately, we haven't actually changed at our core – but our lived experiences have coloured and filtered our natural state of being, layering that childhood version of self with the emotions of life in a world that often feels like a full throttle assault on the senses.

So it can be really useful to drop back into our childhood selves to remember how we landed in this lifetime, what inherent energy we brought, how our natural vibration showed up without any other influences, embodying our own beautiful score of frequency and flow.

Is it coincidental that curiosity, openness and a deeper connection to the natural world tend to be universal themes that we all recognise in our childhood mirror?

One of the most potent benefits of sound healing is its ability to rewire us back into our natural rhythm, to help us become more at home in our bodies, our emotions and our lives simply by operating in our optimal selves. I think that sound healing feels like being gently re-tuned, to your own innate melody.

Take some time to explore for yourself, reconnecting with your natural untainted energy using the 'What's Your Natural Tuning?' exercise that follows. Once you have completed the exercise, it's the perfect time to listen to a sound bath track or practice with your own singing bowls or other instruments, if you have them.

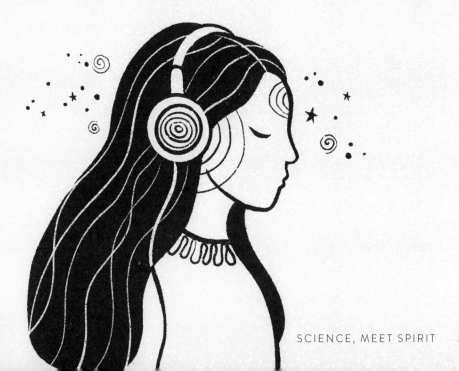

What's Your Natural Tuning?

This is a multi-modal exercise to help you connect with your childhood self, and your natural, untainted energy. Find yourself a quiet space, and have your journal ready, along with your favourite music streaming service.

Read through the exercise in full so you can gather what you need, and then keep your eyes closed unless you are using a photograph as an anchor (see below).

> Take a few deep breaths, and if you have a meditation practice you like, you could start there to bring yourself into stillness. If not, just give yourself a few cycles of simple 4-4-8 breath:

> Inhale through the nose to the count of four.

> Hold your breath at the top of your inhale, to the count of four.

> Exhale slowly through the lips, to the count of eight.

> Recognise that initially, the eight-count may feel challenging. If you run out of air, just keeping counting and set the intention to be measured and slow with the next inhale. Your exhales WILL extend. This is a really helpful conscious breath practice to help bring yourself out of anxiety and help you drop into the influence of the parasympathetic nervous system. I usually use it before a sound journey, to help optimise the experience.

> After 5 or 6 rounds, let your breath drop back into its natural rhythm and notice the easefulness with which you are now inhaling and exhaling. If you sense that your breath is speeding back up, come back to the 4-4-8 pattern for a few more cycles.

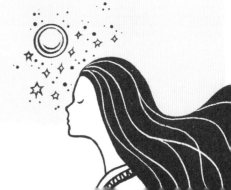

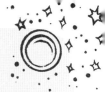

Let's move into a visualisation.

› What comes to mind when you think about your earliest childhood memory?

› Take a beat to find yourself in a visualisation of this experience. If you find visualisation a challenge, you could use a photograph to anchor your awareness and drop you into a specific time and place. Hold the photo in your hand or directly in front of your eyeline and stay focused on it.

› Notice which house and room you are in. Or are you outdoors? Who is there? What do they smell like? If possible, introduce that scent into your space now. What is the backdrop – cars, buildings, furniture, plants, environment. How is the weather? If it's raining, can you simulate that with a soundtrack? Build as full a picture as you can, taking your time.

› Now tune into what you can hear inside your visual. Can you identify sounds, voices, music, sounds from nature? You might like to find an appropriate track to play, bringing your visual to life. For example, I often choose a record I remember my parents playing on our hi-fi when I was very small – something like Queen, Fleetwood Mac or Abba. I've also searched out theme tunes and jingles from TV and radio shows from the early 1980s.

› Go exploring – project yourself back into that younger version of self and take a look around your inner world. What did that day look and feel like from your child's eye perspective? Maybe flashes of memory will bounce into your peripheral vision.

› What words come up for you? They might be descriptive, such as emotions, or tactile experiences such as the fur of a pet, the texture of grass underfoot, or the fabric of clothes or furniture. Do you need to add any more sounds, or change the music accompanying your image? Perhaps you'll put together a short playlist of music and ambient sounds for the next time you practice this exercise.

> Notice if you associate a feeling with your visual. What comes up organically? Peace? Boredom? How is your sense of time? How was life before experiences like pressure, grief, loneliness, confusion, low self-esteem, or failure? Can you project back to who you were before someone broke your heart, you struggled with acceptance at school, or you lost someone important to you? What did the simplicity of human experience feel like, before the world began to tell you who you should be?

> What did the you in your visual like doing – were you a quieter child, did you like to play with animals or catch bumble bees in jars? Did you climb trees or enjoy the wind in your hair when riding a bike, or did you skateboard too fast? Did you talk to people easily, or were you more comfortable with the friends you talked to in your own mind?

> You might want to journal about things you enjoyed at this young age, or about what arises for you from plugging into this young version of yourself. Over time you may find that the visual becomes so comfortable that you can start to roll it back and find an even earlier one.

Bringing It All Together

Let's fast-forward to the present. It seems obvious but is worth saying in capital letters that our natural human state has become influenced, driven by and inherently inverted by stress, a 40-hour week, commuting, phones, the internet, constant blue light, eternal humming from all our devices, the national grid, a disconnection from seasonal cycles and lunar flow, the stresses of young kids, ageing parents, the cost of living and for many of us, a real struggle to be in nature in any tangible way at all.

Is it surprising that we have forgotten how to BE, how to listen to our own vibration, to move to the beat of our own internal drum?

It's nobody's fault. Well, perhaps the guy who came up with the 40-hour working week can shoulder a bit of the blame. But in our relentless effort to progress, to expand into a state of near permanent creation; humanity conversely seems to have started to regress.

In response, as we move out of a century and a half of obsession with industrial revolution, man-made medicine and chemistry, the modern wellness movement offers an intuitive counterbalance, reaching back through the shrouds of regression and pulling forward the threads of the incredible healing tools that our ancestors had nailed thousands of years ago.

Among them, sound healing. Which on our glossy, high-rise, digital skyline, may seem like a throwback to a time of 45s on vinyl and the vintage-hued hippie culture of Glastonbury or Woodstock in decades passed.

But I'm here to ask you to put down that instinctive judgement, because in this new world we can now fuel sound healing with intelligence drawn from its more slick, science-geek sister, sound therapy. This provides a clean landing for soundwork in the world we live in NOW, bringing it bang up to date for the digital 21st century universe.

The sonic siblings – healing and therapy – are separate yet eternally intertwined.

Remember at the beginning of this chapter I referred to them as sides A and B of the old Gen X cassette format? Let's upgrade and consider these twin sonic superpowers to be the original and deluxe editions of today's streamed releases: the same ancient tools humanity has always known about, but remastered for the present.

The places where cosmic sound healing and targeted sound therapy meet and hang out are the corridors of the mind, engineered by the frequency of our brainwaves. In the next chapter we'll look specifically at the impact of sound on the body and in more detail at the super-powered impact of dialling brainwaves up and down using our sound tools.

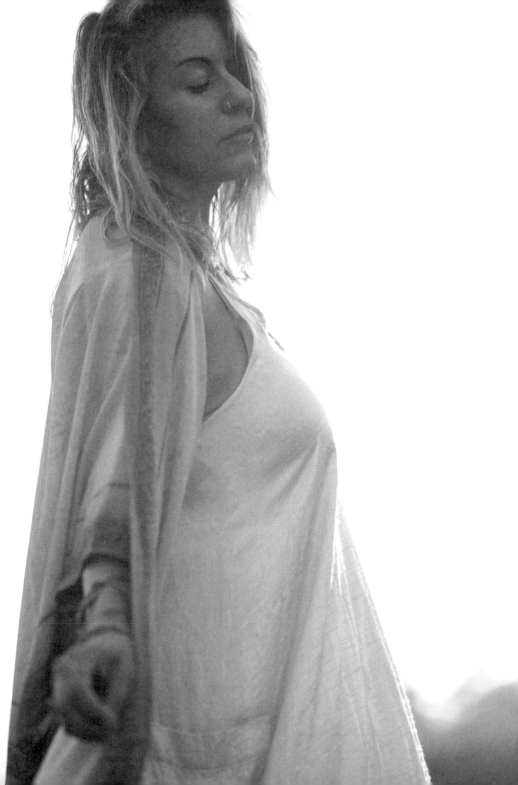

CHAPTER 3

Your Body is a Soundsystem

" It has been found that musical vibrations make their impact upon the entire body, being picked up by the nerves, spinal column, and even by the bones – music affects the pulse, respiration, and blood pressure; but its deepest effects, and those from which most of its curative properties are derived, are mental and emotional." Doren Antrim (Music is Medicine)

The body is a speaker, an amp, and a microphone all at once. With a heck of a lot of cables.

I often introduce sound healing by explaining that the process of feeling sound is a sacred conversation between what's going on outside the body, and the 37 trillion cells inside your physical form.

Yes, 37 trillion cells.

Every last one of them coded with your own unique DNA, and in constant communication with different aspects of your physical, emotional and mental self through the electrical vibrations that allow information to pass in and out of each and every one of those tiny troopers.

Just think of the almost infinite number of micro-transactions going on between your cells in any moment, as your consciousness moves through space and time in this incredible vessel it has chosen for the journey of life. Kind of like a zoomed out Matrix-movie-moment where you can see every single conversation happening on TikTok simultaneously.

Isn't your body INCREDIBLE?

Here's a little context.

When sound is projected into the body, it kicks off an auditory process as the soundwaves bounce through the architecture of our ears. The sonic codes that the inner ear processes are sent into the brain via the auditory nerve (a superhighway trunk road for sound and music) as electrical pulses, which show up neurologically as vibrations. These vibrations get pumped through a kind of Google Translate for the brain, which converts them from electrical Morse code into language. Miraculously the brain also manages to interpret the correct actual language, tone of voice, emotional mood and context as it delivers the message to the conscious part of our brain for our response.

The fact that our bodies have this incredible process for funnelling audible sound into the body blows my mind every time I think about it.

But that's just the beginning because – as we already know to be the magical truth – what we HEAR is only part of the story. Remember, only a fraction of the myriad cells in the body are concerned with hearing in the way we expect. The body can hear through the skin, through bones, and through vibrations that are outside the bounds of human ears (20-20,000Hz), but which we perceive through FEELING rather than hearing.

> Try it out now. With both feet firmly into the floor, notice any vibrations that are arriving in your body through something other than your ears – you could pop your noise cancelling headphones on to test this out more deeply, or refer back to the listening exercise in chapter one for a refresher.

It's through this ability to bring sound into the body in a non-audible way that we FEEL sound as well as HEAR it. It's how the incredible percussionist Evelyn Glennie is able to play instruments even though she is profoundly deaf. It's why you often feel the rumble of thunder way before the bolt of lightning lights up your eyeballs and you actually hear its noise. It's why I always play my gongs in bare feet. Our human bodies are just giant microphones, or maybe amplifiers, conducting sound in a mesmerising symphony in every beat of every breath, in every cell.

So we know that we are wired to experience sound in 360 glorious degrees, but once inside our bodies, where do all those soundwaves physically GO?

Here's the part I really love.

Depending on the nature of the soundwave and the matter it's moving through in your body, you'll notice a kind of rollercoaster effect as the sound hurtles through the dense diamond-like molecular structure of our bones, meanders glacially through the fluid watery texture of our blood, plasma and lymph, and then takes it's sweet, sweet time with the spaces in between, the air and gas.

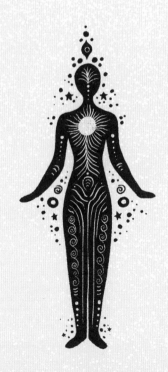

A Watery Soundcheck

To get a sense of how sounds moves through matter in different
ways, take yourself on a sonic adventure... in your bathroom.
This is a good exercise to do next time you have a bath.

To prepare, think of a chorus of a song you really like. If you know
the words that's great, but you could also just hum or overtone
the tune, or just listen on a speaker if you prefer.

1. Start by assessing your bathroom. It's likely to be pretty much all hard
surfaces, but if you do have any soft textures in there like bathmats
or towels, remove them for now. Take any plants out too.

2. Practice your song – sing in your regular voice and notice any
echo or sense of sound bouncing around the room.

3. If you have a bath, start to fill it and sing again. Does
the presence of water change anything?

4. Bring the towels and plants back in, if you had to remove any. When you
start to sing/listen again you'll probably notice these solid structures
act as buffers, diffusing the bouncing sound by absorbing echoes.

5. Finally, once in the bath, practice a submersion test. Play music from a
speaker or your phone, and notice how it sounds with your head fully out of
the water, slightly submerged (so your ears are close to the surface but still
above it), and fully submerged (head and ears under water). How does the
sound differ? What else can you hear? Does it seem high or low in pitch?

Do you notice how the presence of water changes how sound travels?

Remember your body is roughly 60% water.

You can also try this in a swimming pool or the sea – I love to listen
to the sounds of pebbles on the sea bed when floating in the ocean.
You can't hear them at all from the beach, but as soon as you get
under the surface the sonic seascape changes completely.

INPUT CHANNELS – WHERE YOUR VIBES COME FROM

Here's a little reminder – as we come up for a big lungful of clearing air – sound healing is about what's going on OUT THERE, and IN HERE, and how those two processes are interacting.

We are all made of frequencies, so it's pretty logical to state that projecting sound into matter is going to disrupt those frequencies in some way – imagine dropping a pebble into a pond, or skimming it across the surface, if you've got the skills. Test this in a puddle or at home in the kitchen sink and observe just how much the ripples move and evolve. Now visualise that pebble as a sound dropping into your body.

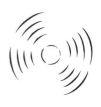

> In liquids, those ripples – vibrations – are pushing matter out of the way as they progress.

> In air or gases, they will completely displace it.

> In solid structures like bones or bricks, sometimes there is an elasticity to the matter and it bounces back once the sound has passed by. Kind of like a giant sonic body check.

> We also all have our own fundamental frequency, and all our organs have their own individual frequencies too. It's a positive symphony in there, and when we send sound vibrations into our body, the existing frequencies respond as if opening the door to a house party, rising and falling to meet and harmonise with the sounds that are passing through. This process is called RESONANCE.

So there's a lot going on both inside and outside the body as we move with soundwaves, whether that movement is throwing shapes on a light-up disco-checked dance floor or lying in the long grass in the summer sunshine, listening to the ocean waves.

But that's not all – we are also affected by vibrations created by other people's energy. We all know how uncomfortable it feels to walk into the dinner party kitchen where the hosts have just been gloves-off in a colossal argument. Or that uneasy tingle down our spines that shows up when we hear the voice of someone we don't especially want to see or connect with. RESONANCE works in reverse too, showing us what dis-harmony feels like.

Other vibrations that can alter the sound of our own natural state of being include man-made structures that create physical blocks. Think about your internet router at home – the more walls are between it and your laptop, the less good your connection. Highly charged chunky heavyweights such as cars, concrete buildings or even objects that carry a lot of their own frequency, like big electrical machines or broadband boxes, could all manifest as barriers that stop your natural frequency from being connected with or felt clearly.

To be clear – I'm not saying you should stay away from all these things. The internet certainly has its uses! And I for one have tried and failed to give up the smartphone hustle countless times. Participation in the civilisation we live in demands connection – but we can still apply awareness, especially now we know that all matter vibrates and is in conversation with your own cells.

So just be careful where you put your energy, ok?

And remember that this is why sound studios, concert halls and theatres always have strange looking spongy shapes all over the ceilings, tons of heavy drapes and carpets from a different dimension. Never checked? Don't do yourself out of a glance up and down next time, especially in those amazing 1960s buildings – it's fascinating, sonically-informed interior design.

So what this all adds up to is a simple natural law, one which runs the game on the subtle vibratory connection between cells in our bodies, and the exchange of microcosmic energetic information between us and what or whoever else is around us.

It's called the LAW OF ENTRAINMENT, and it's coming your way. Notebooks at the ready for some really, REALLY cool science.

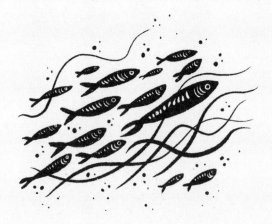

SCIENCE CLASS: THE LAW OF ENTRAINMENT

Entrainment is one of nature's most powerful modes – a fundamental law of physics, having being noted and named in 1665 by physicist Christian Huygens, himself a force of nature who contributed groundbreaking findings to the field of classical mechanics. His work on telescopes and lenses has gifted modern astronomy most of the science on which its viewing instruments rely – oh and his DIY telescopes were so slick, he even discovered Saturn's main moon Titan with one. By accident.

Huygens also invented the pendulum clock – in its day the most accurate timekeeper ever created, and in the course of his development of the futuristic timepiece he established the principle of ENTRAINMENT.

The basic principle of entrainment is that when two different frequencies are in each other's presence, they will always move into resonance with each other; the lower frequency will move up to meet the higher one in a process we call synchronicity.

It's natural harmony.

The Law of Entrainment can be seen across many areas and aspects of science, music and nature. Huygens first saw it in action when he realised two adjacent pendulum clocks that were initially pulsing at different speeds naturally came into resonance with each other over a period of time.

We see the same principle in murmurations of starlings, in the way shoals of fish manage to stay in beautiful synchronicity as they weave through the water, and in fireflies whose wings beat in unison to create a flashbulb effects as they sit in twilight trees.

The basic science is that the resonance is created by small amounts of energy bouncing between two objects moving at slightly different speeds. The stronger of the two will gradually dominate until the weaker object comes into synchronicity. Together they beat as a pair, and in doing do immediately preserve energy and theoretically at least, create inherent connection.

You know when you walk into a room and see your best friend or the love of your life across the room? THAT connection.

It's easy to see why vibrating in harmony with nature is appealing.

For animals, saving energy through synchronicity means there is more left to pour into their wings and hooves, and also the consistent beat of the group or pack provides clearer audio space for identifying danger. You know this too – because it's hard to listen to instructions over the racket of a crowd, or conversation in the chaos of a family kitchen at 6pm. But if everybody is making the same sound, at the same time, suddenly... space and clarity unfolds.

The circadian rhythms that are fundamental to life are based on this principle too – when we throw our bodyclock out with a late night we disrupt our waking cycle, the one that's synchronised to the path of the Sun. When we get on a plane and fly round the world, we are beating to an entirely different pulse to the place we've landed. That stomach-lurching rollercoaster of jet lag could be said to be entrainment, as our physical body is dragged kicking and screaming into resonance with its new environment.

I also love the example of a football crowd, or very especially, a gig. 90,000 people making different noises is a deafening wall of sound. 90,000 people clapping or singing in unison, and suddenly it all makes sense. You can hear what's happening on the pitch or on stage, and you know WHY you're there. What's more, you can FEEL the resonance of the artist on stage, the crowd around you, the CONNECTION. Ever wonder where home advantage comes from on the sports field? Well, now you know.

Where else in life can you identify entrainment? Between yourself, the people you love, strangers, nature? Try the exercise that follows to identify what this cosmic and yet utterly logical groove truly feels like in your body and in your heart.

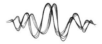

Exploring Entrainment

ANIMAL MAGIC

I especially like cats for this experiment, but any pet or person will do!

Start by checking your own resting heart rate. Do this by counting beats per minute with index and middle fingers taking your pulse at the wrist.

If possible, take the heart rate of your pet or person too.

Come into close connection – maybe curling up on the sofa and bringing your head to the other person's shoulder or chest; or give your cat a good snuggle. My cat used to love lying across my heart, which was optimum for this test!

Simply breathe and be. After 4 or 5 minutes you may notice that your breathing has synchronised or at least come into the same rhythmic pattern as your partner. You can check heart rates again and notice differences – have they entrained?

PLANT POWER

Plants respond to resonance too:

Buy a bunch of fresh flowers and split them in two. Place them in two different areas of your home, with different light levels.

After a couple of days, observe that one is looking a little less lively than the other. Place both bunches in a new, neutral space, next to each other.

Notice how the fading blooms resonate, and adjust to appear the same as their neighbours once again.

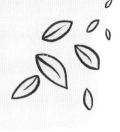

So back to SOUND HEALING, because entrainment is not just for the science lab – it's also a fundamental pillar of the musical world.

I love to work with the shamanic drum in my sessions – and when we talk about instruments later on we'll get into more of the musical and spiritual detail on why this is. But a core contribution the drum makes from the scientific perspective is to create a beat, a rhythm, for every guest in the soundspace to entrain to. It's a pacemaker that brings the room into resonance – with the drum, with me, and with each other. In such a receptive state, the stage is set for the self-healing journey described in chapter two to truly begin.

Led by the visionary Dr Joe Dispenza, the Heartmath Institute in California has conducted detailed studies on entrainment between people. Dr Dispenza (but hey, you can call him Dr Joe) leads the way in the research that explores the links between neuroscience and physiological function with healing modalities and meditation. The rock star researchers involved with these studies talk about "helping to demystify the impact of the mind on the body" and it's mind-blowing work. Literally.

The Heartmath Institute has now established that when various systems of the body become entrained to the HEART, the body moves into a new "physio-emotional" state that facilitates optimised healing. They rather sexily call this phenomenon 'heart coherence'.

In this state, according to their research, our bodily systems function as if on some kind of natural rocket fuel, spiking in efficiency while amplifying and igniting our inherent healing capacity. The team suggest that overall health and consciousness benefits of heart coherence include "reduced stress, anxiety and depression; decreased burnout and fatigue; enhanced immunity and hormonal balance; improved cognitive performance and enhanced learning; increased organizational effectiveness; and health improvements in a number of clinical populations".

The Heartmath Institute and other sound science experts have pointed out that entrainment happens across all scales of existence. On a micro scale, it's happening at a subatomic level across every tiny molecule of the material universe; and simultaneously some of the biggest objects in the galaxy – planets, for example – are also dancing with each other, finding resonance. There's plenty of mind-bending and fascinating storytelling and research that places orbital entrainment as integral to the history of our solar system – with giant Jupiter's pulling of every other pile of rubble in the region into his own rhythm said to be a huge part of how life ended up flourishing on this third rock from the Sun. Just ask rockstar-physicist Professor Brian Cox.

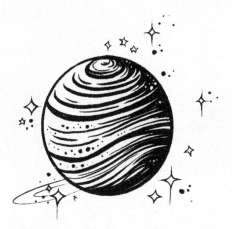

But when it comes to working in the soundspace, what we need to take away from this fascinating trawl – from a couple of 17th century clocks to heavy meditators hooked up to EKG machines in millennial California – is that NATURE LOVES HARMONY.

Nature shows us repeatedly that life was built to be in resonance. It's the secret source of connection.

Sound healing can plug us into that place of resonance, so that we too are participating in a resonant world of health and harmony.

When we lie in a sound bath (nope, no bathing suit required) our environment becomes a wash of soundwaves selected specifically by your sound healer or facilitator for their high vibration and ability to bring us out of our potentially toxic and exhausted states of body and mind. We begin to entrain to the new frequencies soaring through our cells. Our heart and brain adapt and synchronise their frequency to match what is being projected into the space, the body and its biofield.

We begin to ascend: euphoria, a natural high, a sense of perfect alignment, everything in its right place, being present in absolutely the right time. It's such a rare and juicy moment when we feel completely at ease with life. We've all felt it, in those spaces where a group collectively elevates – perhaps in a kundalini yoga class, in the golden circle at a gig, at the last wedding you went to.

This natural harmony is available to us all in the soundspace. Absolute bliss, complete balance, perfect resonance.

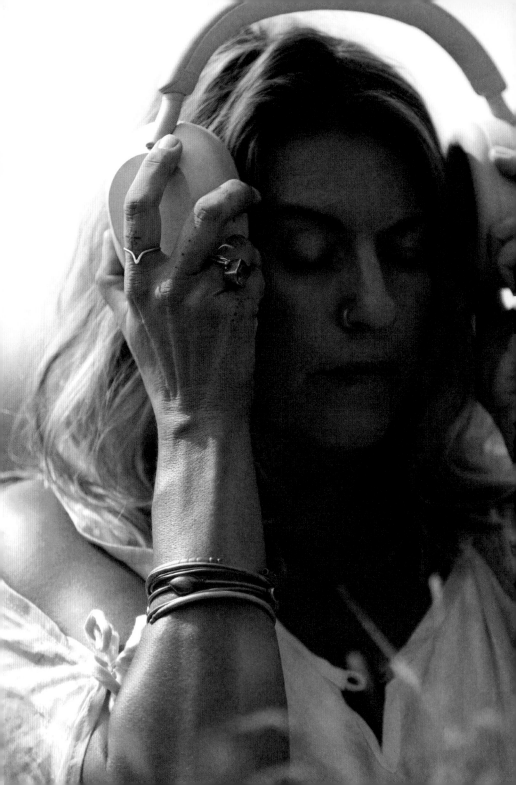

CHAPTER 4
Inside the Binaural Beatbox

"*Everything is energy. Match the frequency of the reality you want and you cannot help but get that reality. It can be no other way. This is not philosophy. This is physics.*" Albert Einstein, Nobel prize physicist

If your body is a soundsystem, then your BRAIN is your synthesiser.

It can literally create and modulate almost anything.

Your brain is the supercomputer that runs it all. Since the dawn of modern medicine, the smartest minds have been trying to work out exactly what goes on in our grey matter, and they can still only account for around 3% of it. Meaning that there is a LOT of scope for learning, expanding, and pushing out the edges of what we think we know about how our consciousness functions.

But here's some great stuff we DO know about the black box of our mind.

The human brain has its own array of frequency bands, brainwave states at which it operates in a prismatic, expansive array of levels. Moving between brainwave states allows us to tap into a deep reservoir of different shapes of being. Want to drop into one of those luscious, log-like 12 hour sleeps that only students seem able to achieve naturally? There's a frequency for that. Got to write a proposal or pitch in the next hour and need to tap into Steve Jobs-style vision? There's a frequency for that too.

Sound healing is the most potent and powerful way of reaching into the brain's mainframe and manually twirling the graphic equalizers of our mind. In doing so, we entrain our brain to the desired frequency in the same way we would tune an old-style radio (think 1980s transistor), nudging and easing the dial until it comes into alignment with the frequency on which the signal is being transmitted, thus delivering... sound. And not just sound, but SPECIFIC HEALING FREQUENCIES. Boom!

Your brain has five key brainwave states. There are a few more, if you want to get into serious white coat knowledge, but for the purposes of sound healing, these are the inner radio stations of your mind:

Gamma (40-80Hz)

SUPERHUMAN SKILLS

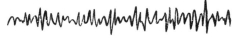

Great for... Intense focus, memory recall, deep compassion, hyper-visualisation

Beta (13-40Hz)

THE DAILY GRIND

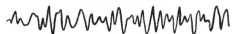

Great for... Mental alertness, cognitive activity, sensory perception

Alpha (8-12Hz)

COOL, CALM, COLLECTED

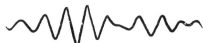

Great for... Creative learning, singular focus, relaxation and tunnel vision

Theta (4-7Hz)

KALEIDOSCOPE CONSCIOUSNESS

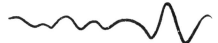

Great for... Visual meditation, hypnosis, trance state, supraconsciousness, dream state

Delta (0.5-3Hz)

EXTREME REST

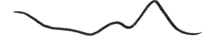

Great for... Deep sleep, profound healing, loss of bodily awareness, non-duality

Let's do a chart rundown of the top five.

The Gamma brainwave is a hyper-cognitive state that we don't spend much time in – in fact for the longest time, scientists didn't even have the equipment to measure brain frequencies at this level, believing the 25Hz was the fastest our brains could cycle! Our senses are usually too busy firing a barrage of information at us for our overwhelmed minds to be able to stay in this supercomputer state for long – unless we happen to be an elite athlete or iconic performer, both of whom are known to flourish in gamma state and are said to have a naturally higher occurring level of these superwaves.

Gamma is mostly consistent with peak performance, incredible memory recall and a laser-like focus that is so intense you might almost feel the tiny cogs of your brain whirring. This is also the state we move towards in the deepest meditations, especially those that work with compassion and empathy at their heart. I call it the master meditator frequency. The monks in Tibet have this down.

In our usual waking day we are operating in Beta brainwave, where our five functional senses feed the brain and we manage to get from A to B based on practicality and physical coordination. Our senses keep us safe – my favourite anecdote about Beta brain action is that without it we'd seriously struggle to move through the 3D world without bodychecking ourselves on every door frame. For a start, we'd all be looking at the end of our noses and hitting the deck on a daily basis. Sound strange? Our brains are constantly feeding us a whole bunch of illusory content to help keep us in our human lane, and Beta brainwave is where this high functioning skillset flourishes. This is where we get our lives lived and our to-do lists smashed out.

As our brainwaves slow down a little more, we arrive in Alpha state. This is definitely more relaxed than Beta simply because our window of focus dramatically narrows. Yogis may recognise this state as close to dharana or dhyana, a stillpoint place of clarity, with less distraction in the peripheral vision. It's an optimum state for studying and locking into something you might call 'flow state' or constructive rest, where your brain is busy with just one primary task. In the soundspace, I usually find that people are down to a single active sense in alpha state, and it's often scent – known to be the first sensory attunement we connect with at birth, and the last one the brain recognises before death. Alpha is kind of like racehorse blinkers for your brain, or driving a car with no mirrors dragging your gaze outwards – it's the state I'm in right now as I write these words!

As we drop down into Theta brainwave, this is where things start to get really interesting. Which is rather ironic, as the brainwave itself is beginning to flatten out in this slow-motion kaleidoscopic state. It's in my script to remind all comers to the soundspace that this brainwave state is where many of the world's creative geniuses were, or are, believed to reside at least semi-permanently – from Picasso to Beethoven, Keith Richards to Kurt Cobain. For anyone looking to expand their creative consciousness, this is the place to hang out and be free.

Here in the shadowlands, our functional senses have left the building and we can connect to the aspects of the mind that exist in that hazy 97% of unknown. We'll be diving into this liminal state in our deeper exploration of expanded consciousness, but this languid brainwave vibration – also reached with many plant medicines and opioids – is known to be a place where the mirrors of our mind can take a deliciously psychedelic turn.

Here, the veil between form and consciousness is sheer to non-existent, and ALL experiences are on the table, from observable vision-like imagery to clarion-clear internal voices, messages from spirit and channelled wisdom.

Theta brainwave has long been associated with powerful creativity – I've seen so many guests over the years arrive back from a sound journey and become immediately compelled, obsessed almost, with the desire to draw, write and scribble down the visionary ideas that have landed for them while in the helter-skelter of the Theta mind.

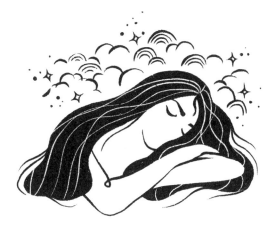

Finally, dreamy Delta. A brainwave so slow and horizontal it's almost comatose. Literally.

In these most glacial of frequencies, the human brain has left the building and is closing the door behind it. In Delta state we can experience a level of rest so far beyond what we achieve in our blue-lit, distorted nightly sleep, that it's hard to imagine that we function without it. The physical body is almost completely switched off, the messaging system from the brain to the muscles and nerves is at total rest. Not on standby, in the way we turn our TVs off at night and leave that persistent red light on. OFF. Unplugged at the wall. Master reset.

Delta state offers us such a deep regeneration that when our brainwaves stay here, we can receive the cellular equivalent of around five hours of sleep in just 40 minutes. It's the ultimate hustle-culture bypass. In Delta, our bodies can 'disappear' – we are SO deeply out of our regular functional state that sometimes we have the feeling of either sinking through the floor or levitating off into space. The choice is yours, and intention will be your guide as it signposts your odyssey through dreamland.

Either way, our consciousness is very much absent and deep Delta often drops us into a cosmic conversation with non-duality – that supreme sense of one-ness. Often guests suspect or worry they have fallen asleep when Delta hits (trust me when I say there is NO sound I haven't heard in the soundspace, including surround-sound snoring!) and while it's true that in some of our nightly deep sleep we do get to this stage occasionally, being guided into and supported in this state during a curated sound immersion offers a totally different Delta experience.

So how do we actually get the dials moving, to control our brainwaves, and access these powerful healing, regenerative, and meditative states?

There are a few ways. For some you may need my help, but plenty are DIY. Brainwave entrainment is like a workout for your grey matter. By harnessing its inherent plasticity and finessing the frequency, we can ALL tap into our self-healing power through sound.

In a sound bath, sound journey, soundscape – whatever phrasing your trusty local sound practitioner has selected to market their services – you just need to bring yourself and your intention. Your facilitator is there to project sounds into the forcefield of the environment, flooding your body and biofield with the perfect combination of frequencies.

In some cases, simply cultivating a wall of sonic vibration is enough, as most sound healing instruments organically activate Theta and Delta brainwaves to some degree. Particularly for therapeutic applications, very specific frequencies will be selected – for example, I use precisely chosen tuning forks to create specific brainwave frequencies for my clients. In group sound odysseys (that's the descriptor I go with and I love its liquid-like connotations) I like to build a true point-to-point journey through the way I construct my sessions, and consciously move guests through the brainwave states with my choice of sound tools and verbal guidance.

But one of the easiest ways to access your own brainwave controls is through your favourite streaming service.

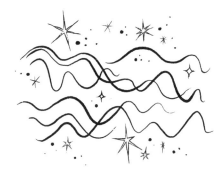

Working with Binaural Beats

Headphones are essential so grab yours now, along with your journal.

This is a half hour exercise, so make space in your day and ensure your environment is distraction-free.

Start the playlist and for the first few minutes, bring yourself into a receptive state by practicing the conscious 4-4-8 breathwork we've used before (see Chapter 2, What's Your Natural Tuning?)

The playlist will take you on a guided journey through Alpha, Theta and Gamma brainwaves, before easing you into a longer Delta rest.

At the end of the playlist, grab your journal and respond to the following prompts:

1. What feels really clear for me right now?

2. Can I identify a singular idea or project that I know needs my attention?

3. Are some new, unusual or unexpected ideas or themes surfacing? Take time to sit with this and notice even the smallest flicker of something outside of your current projects, plans or awareness. It might feel totally leftfield or confusing so remain OPEN.

4. Do I feel more aware of particular colours, scents or shapes? Sit for a moment to consider this.

5. How is my body? Do I feel heavier or lighter? Did any parts of my body feel as if they vanished or disappeared during the sound journey? Do I feel as if I have been asleep?

Remember to drink plenty of water and stretch a little before you plug back into your day. It's great to get bare feet into grass or earth if you can. You could also put on some sounds to encourage Beta brainwaves to bring your conscious/functional senses back online.

BINAURAL BEATS: YOUR PERSONAL MIXING DESK

BINAURAL BEATS are having a zeitgeist moment, and why shouldn't they? When you realise just how potent these easy-access tracks can be in supporting our wellbeing, healing and mental health, it seems like an untapped open goal not to have them on pretty much all the time.

So what exactly IS a binaural beat?

It's an aural illusion. It sounds complex, but like everything sound-healing-related, it's brilliantly simple when you peel back the layers and look at the basics.

Working with binaural beats means specifically playing two different sounds into your ears, one each side. For this reason, if you want to truly nail DIY sound healing it's really important to have a pair of headphones on when you listen to binaural beats. It's not that you can't enjoy the sounds themselves through speakers, but directly controlling brainwaves does require a little bit of tech. But just a little – any stereo headphones will do. Even your vintage Sony Walkman ones.

When binaural beats tracks have been crafted and mastered by a properly trained audio magician they will be delivered in a way that the sound playing into your right headphone is just a little different to what's pumping through the left. This is absolutely FUNDAMENTAL to how the whole experience works.

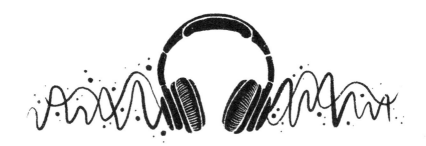

Cue the science. The two frequencies played into each ear are specifically selected to be a certain number of hertz (Hz) apart. When the brain receives the two signals simultaneously it turns into a sound engineer and creates a third tone – which is the difference between the two original sounds.

It's this third tone that the brain hears and entrains to.

So if one ear receives a frequency of 200Hz and the other receives 210Hz, the difference of 10Hz is what the brain processes. 10Hz is an ALPHA brainwave, and just like that, you're in charge of your brainwave frequencies and deciding in which state you want and need to be operating right now.

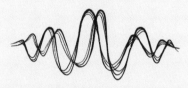

The world – or at least the online sound community – is your oyster. Just think how much more efficient you can be while studying or writing your book, how much more quickly you can fall into truly restful, regenerative sleep, or how much more benefit you can get from your morning meditation practice, whether it's sitting in your living room or squished up on the tube on your daily commute.

You've just touched the power of sound healing. How does it feel?

Now you know all about the incredible scalability and megapower of our brainwaves, you can marry up that knowledge with the entrainment theory we discussed in the previous chapter. This intersectional meeting of science and spirit brings us full circle to the HEALING POWER OF SOUND.

Pretty cool huh?

MAKING SENSE OF THE 3D WORLD

That's a pretty deep dive into the black box of the brainwave. So let's talk about how our brain receives physical, sensory information that also feeds into the sound healing landscape.

Our brilliant bodies run predominantly on the messages received by our five functional senses – our eyes, ears, nose, tongue and fingertips all play a pivotal role in collecting information about what's happening in our biofield and beyond. They deliver their findings to the post room of our mind as sensory perception, alerting us to danger, joy, opportunity – the full bandwidth of human emotions.

Or so we think.

The five functional senses – what we see, hear, taste, touch and smell, are fantastic tools to help us get through life. Organically, they are perfectly tuned to our needs – a fact illuminated even more by just how much we feel impeded when one of them starts to misfire. For example, losing our sense of smell was something collectively experienced to unseen levels during the pandemic of 2020-2022. For the many millions of people faced with no sense of smell for the first time in their lives, experiencing a fragrance-free world became a strangely disembodied experience. Likewise, the midlife moment where you suddenly realise that your vision is beginning to give you a distorted perspective can create an uncharted sense of vulnerability.

So our five senses – let's call them the 3D senses – keep us moving through the world safely and with all the intel we need to hunt, gather and nurture. In the modern day that looks like getting us to the supermarket safely, allowing us to drive, and helping us decipher the endless collection of appliances in our kitchens. Although not quite everybody has that part nailed, of course!

But it would be misleading to think these are the ONLY senses we have, or need.

Buried in that 97% of unmapped mindscape, we have a myriad of other senses – I like to call them the ETHERIC, or 5D senses. It's through these that we can pick up experiences, messages, and intelligent insight from somewhere other than the immediate physical landscape.

And THESE are the senses that allow us to move beyond the forests of the conscious mind, places often overwhelmed, overworked and over-stimulated; and into the eternal oceans of what lies beyond the body we see on scans, x-rays and with our eyes; the unconscious, subconscious, or supra-conscious mind. You might have experienced this aspect of self in your dreams, in that twilight state after a long night on the dance floor, or perhaps in your savasana – that long lie down at the end of a yoga class that is the secret reason everyone is really on the mat at all.

Think about when you can most easily drop out of your day-to-day mental chaos. When can you finally tune out the grinding to-do lists, the struggle to remember to put fuel in the car while worrying about your energy bill and the mental health mist snapping at your heels?

When your senses are lowered, or off. That's when. Have you ever experienced a flotation tank? It's a sensory deprivation chamber where, in the darkness and silence, floating in the saltiest water to keep you from touching the sides, you become unplugged from the relentless messaging pouring into the mind. Why do you think most meditations begin with a cue to 'softly let your eyes flutter to a close...'? The entire physical purpose of the lotus posture in yoga is to close off the senses, and the energetic channels that act as pathways into the body.

Without our five functional senses taking up all the bandwidth, we can really start to connect with the other senses and portals in and out of our body. This is where that full body listening I've been coaching you towards can really take flight.

Now that we know that entrainment creates harmony, and harmony is our optimum state of being for healing, therapeutic effectiveness, and for generally being in a pretty juicy groove, we want to GET THERE, right?

You've got binaural beats to get your brain entrained.

So now we need to get some physical vibrations and sounds powering through your body, your energetic system, your heart.

It's time to pick up your instruments, and PLAY.

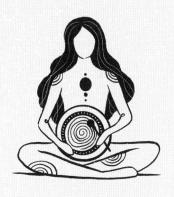

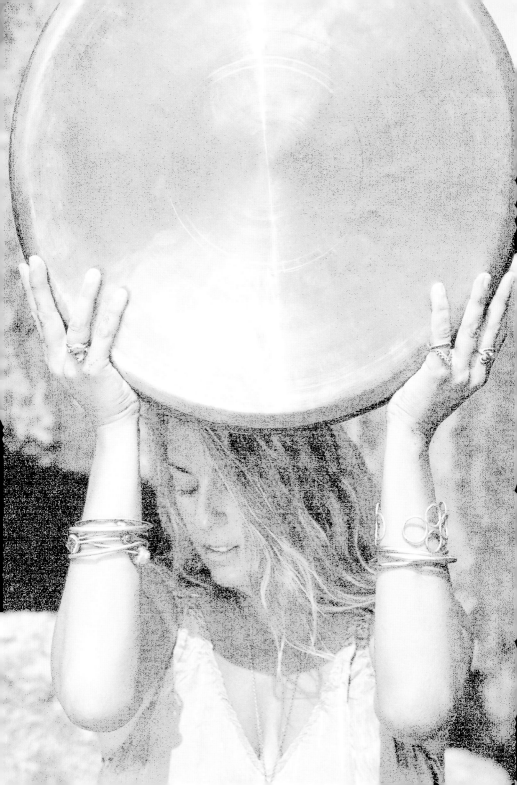

CHAPTER 5
Time to Press Play

"Emotions of any kind can be evoked by melody and rhythm; therefore music has the power to form character." Aristotle, philosopher and polymath

When did you last pick up a musical instrument?

Have you EVER played one? Let me guess – you can knock out a couple of tunes on the recorder, right? Or you can bash out 'chopsticks' on the piano. It's a stone cold classic.

And it all counts. Just like the triangle, the tambourine, and banging a drum count. Music isn't always reading a score or making like Jimi Hendrix on those complex chords. I'm not for a second saying that musicality isn't fundamental to sound healing, in fact I believe deeply that it is, and I'll tell you why later on. However, it's a fact that you don't need to be able to play an instrument to participate, create or benefit from sound healing.

I read a something on the internet (and that's as reliable a source as I have) which is utterly impossible to quantify but feels like it has potential resonance with a lot of people. I want to see how it makes you feel, so here it is:

20% of kids learn to play music, and 70% of adults wish they had.

Well true or not, it's never too late. The great news is that so many instruments that you'll see in the soundspace are very simple to learn and bring into your own home with ease. Not to entirely diminish my own skills, or that of the many other extensively trained sound healing facilitators out there in the cosmos, because to do this work WELL, with creativity, artfulness and authenticity (yes, it's buzzword time again), to make a profound energetic and evolutionary impact on people is far more than just clattering instruments with abandon. And it's certainly not just about intuition, although that too is vital to the sounds we make.

Sound healing instruments are infinitely more accessible than you think, even to the adults who secretly wish they hadn't spent music class gazing out of the window. Perhaps that's partly why there is such a proliferation of new sound artists, healers, practitioners and therapists out there, picking up where they left off in their youth.

Let's take a look at the instruments you'll see in the sound healing space, and discover how you can connect with them yourself in both receptivity and creativity.

Don't forget – what the science of sound has taught us is that we are ALL music, all vibration, and the world IS sound. You just need to start playing.

"Teach the student first, the music second, and the piano third."

Frances Clark, pianist, teacher and academic

The architecture of sound healing is crafted from an array of instruments.

In most western iterations of the sound bath, you'll see some combination of gongs and singing bowls. Some practitioners specialise in one or the other, some – and I'm sticking my neck out to say these tend to be the ones with a more naturally musical background – integrate both, and bring multiple different instruments into a session.

You might encounter a culturally familiar collection of instruments that is reminiscent of the orchestra pit or the stage kit at a music festival, perhaps laced with a peculiar bunch of oddities that you've only ever seen in the souks and markets of your holiday travels, or shoved in a corner at the charity/thrift shop.

Many players incorporate stringed instruments such as the classical harp, acoustic guitar, monochord, or Persian santur. A more shamanic sound bath might involve various drums, flutes and rattles. If your practitioner doubles up as a yogi you may notice a harmonium or shruti box – both variations of a small floor-based organ. A more future-focused facilitator may have a synthesiser or mixing desk in their kit, and handpans are definitely having a global moment too.

And is it really a sound bath without a wind chime or two? I doubt it.

The great thing is, any combination of instruments works. When I started playing I used to panic about using EVERY. SINGLE. INSTRUMENT in front of me. It made for an almightily chaotic setup and I'm sure I emptied a good few studios in the early days from my determination to prove what a multi-instrumentalist I was.

In truth, some of my most magical sessions have been delivered with just a couple of singing bowls and a bag of lentils (yes really – all will be revealed!).

Remember that sound healing is about adjusting the frequency and vibration of your body. That said, some instruments are simply better suited to those with a bit of inherent musical experience or a willingness to acquire it. Although gongs and crystal bowls are easy to get a sound out of, it does need a degree of training and musicality to make it a tolerable sound rather than an unholy racket. You still have ears, and taste levels (as do your neighbours, FYI). So making a NICE noise, rather than just white noise, is eminently desirable!

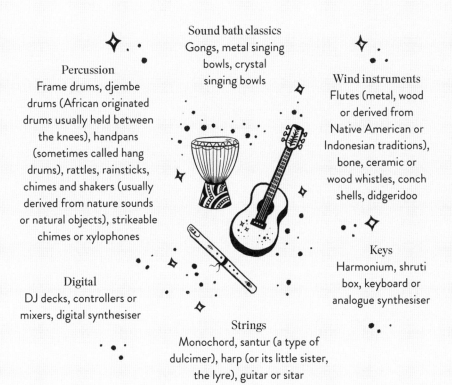

Sound bath classics
Gongs, metal singing bowls, crystal singing bowls

Percussion
Frame drums, djembe drums (African originated drums usually held between the knees), handpans (sometimes called hang drums), rattles, rainsticks, chimes and shakers (usually derived from nature sounds or natural objects), strikeable chimes or xylophones

Wind instruments
Flutes (metal, wood or derived from Native American or Indonesian traditions), bone, ceramic or wood whistles, conch shells, didgeridoo

Digital
DJ decks, controllers or mixers, digital synthesiser

Keys
Harmonium, shruti box, keyboard or analogue synthesiser

Strings
Monochord, santur (a type of dulcimer), harp (or its little sister, the lyre), guitar or sitar

Obviously, this list is FAR from exhaustive and depending on where you are in the world, or the provenance/training of your sound facilitator, you may encounter all kinds of other wonderful instruments.

If you can play the piano to any degree then a harmonium will probably be an easy enough transition. If you can get a few chords out of a guitar or even just have your staple campfire songs (Neil Young? You and me both), then the finger action and coordination of monochords will naturally just make sense. Perhaps like me you played the classical flute as a kid, in which case you definitely have a head start on the traditional wooden and bamboo types.

Reassuringly, plenty of instruments are totally available to anyone who fancies having a go – skills or no skills. It's common knowledge that Paul McCartney has never been able to read music, and Liam Gallagher is ironically noted for his primary instrumental contribution to his band Oasis being a tambourine. Everyone has rhythm and music in their soul, whatever way it shows up in their body.

Getting Started With Sound Healing Instruments

My top tips for bringing sound into your own practice, on an entry level budget and lo-fi musical skills.

› Frame drum: a simple shamanic skinned drum is a great place to start. Practice creating different rhythms and volumes using a beater or your hand. Try singing or overtoning (see Chapter 7, Awakening the Voice) across the surface of the drum.

› Wind chimes: Koshi chimes are so simple and are great way to get started. See if you can hear the seven different tones inside the chime as it moves, isolating them in your mind. Practice moving the chime around your aura and chakras – wafting it slowly about three inches away from the surface of your body – and see what you notice.

› Tongue drum: a kind of hybrid drum and xylophone, metal tongue drums are a great way to get used to scales and chords. Use a mallet in each hand and practice creating and moving between pairs of notes.

Later in this chapter and the next you'll find ideas for small gongs and singing bowls too.

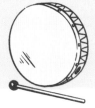

FROM ANCIENT CHINA TO PROG ROCK IN POMPEII – THE STORY OF THE GONG

At one of the very first sound healing sessions I went to – in East London sometime in the mid 00s – I came face to face with what I now know to be the biggest gong in the UK. This particular gong was a light, iridescent golden colour that seemed otherworldly, yet its main feature was undeniably its giant scale. Standing at a lofty diameter of 80 inches and bathed in spotlights and oceanic projections, it looked like the moon, just hanging out in a basement somewhere off Shoreditch High Street.

It sounded like the moon too, or at least how I always imagined the velvet skies of our evocative satellite to sound. A completely cosmic, shimmering and shuddering sound from deep beyond the edges of consciousness, apparently from the molten core of the earth and yet as if it was being beamed in from a civilisation across the galaxy. I recall my mind flickering to the novels and futuristic dreamscapes of Isaac Asimov or the space opera of *2001: A Space Odyssey*. I had no idea of the what, where, how or why of that incredible sound, but I wanted to know more.

Gongs are amongst the most elusive and yet utterly present instruments in the sound healing world. While sound healing encompasses many variations and forms – from singular studies in crystal bowls to bespoke collections of instruments, the ascendance of digital tools and of course, the oldest instrument of all: the human voice – nothing symbolises and, in my view, epitomises a sound healing space as readily as the gong.

Their sheer weight and shine, not to mention gilded price tag, makes these beasts of the soundstage impossible to miss. Originating as far as we know from the caves of what is now Afghanistan and Turkmenistan around 4500 years ago, most musical historians agree that the gong began life as some sort of signalling instrument. I mean, it's a hard sound to miss and would have been extremely handy as a dinner bell on the vast plains of ancient Asia, that's for sure.

Gongs showed up in various cultures and traditions of the Far East over the subsequent centuries, with China, Vietnam, Indonesia and Myanmar emerging as hotspots for gong manufacture and the cultural inclusion of these curious metal discs in theatre, ceremony and the workplace. Even today many countries and communities in this part of the world hold gongs as a key aspect of family life, using them to bring clearing energy to the home in a daily ritual as familiar as the essential morning tea and toast tradition is to England, or making that first coffee of the day.

There are a few places people tend to recognise gongs from: the end of *Bohemian Rhapsody*; dinner gongs on BBC period television dramas; Pink Floyd at Pompeii; that guy banging a gong at the beginning of old Rank films (apparently that one was made of papier-mâché though).

Playable gongs tend to be made of a rather more resilient material. Bronze alloy is a mix of copper and tin, although many gongs also have a sprinkling of zinc and there is an exciting new breed of creative musical artisans working with a fusion of futuristic-sounding metals such as nickel and titanium. The material is fundamental to the sound, with the higher copper content and dash of iron sported by many gongs from the east making them the big beasts of any sound healer's setup. These offer a deeper sonic earthquake than the shinier, prettier western-made gongs that tend to have more mirage-like astral harmonics and a longer sustain.

Guests in my soundspace are always utterly entranced by these curious cosmic disks, wondering what it is they actually DO. For what it's worth, I think that gongs are the gateway to the more transcendent aspects of sound healing, as well as being a primary inducer of the brainwave states that take us into altered consciousness.

The immersive oceanic nature of their sounds is inescapable; they create such an all-consuming sonic landscape that once you're bundled up in your blanket and in their grasp, it's impossible to be anywhere else either mentally or physically. They demand surrender, and as a result they are powerfully effective in creating a space to allow self healing, even in the most hardwired millennial brains and bodies. I so often hear feedback that guests who found themselves locked in a boxing match with their persistent monkey mind during the early stages of a sound journey literally felt the earth move beneath and within them as the gongs transported them out of their bodies and into that deep Theta- and Delta-hued dreamscape.

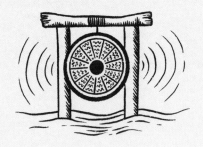

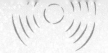

Some gongs are tuned to a fundamental note and frequency, some are not. Lots of gongs are said to be tuned to elemental energies or planetary frequencies – a particularly space-age endeavour pioneered by Swiss number-cruncher Hans Cousto in his 1978 masterpiece of musical mathematics, *The Cosmic Octave*.

A pioneer of the field of psychonautics (the study of altered states of consciousness and how to get there), Cousto worked out some hefty equations to establish the audio frequencies of planets and other galactic bodies. Eagle-eyed gong manufacturers jumped on this alluring meeting of maths and music and began to produce gongs tuned to Cousto's freshly minted planetary frequency table – it was a masterstroke for the sales team, but has it ever really added up to anything other than a gimmick for a gullible New Age?

Actually, I think it has. Disclaimer: I'm an astrologist too, so a gong tuned to the frequency of Saturn is a niche I'm definitely here for. But nonetheless, I have a healthy enough pragmatic streak to always approach this kind of thing with a decent shot of suspicion.

My feeling is that the evidence is best observed in the experience, and my own experience of working with the planetary gongs has been that there truly is a correlation between the transcendent journey of the recipient and the themes of the planetary frequencies. Of course, gongs entrain with each other in the most majestic manner, and I often feel that the interplay and entrainment of two gongs is rooted in the same framework as a transiting aspect in the skies. Coincidence? Maybe. Maybe not.

It's definitely the case that some gongs flutter their eyelids at us while others send us into a spiral leading straight to the door. I've had countless people take one look at my Mercury gong, mutter something about retrogrades and insist that they "don't like that one". Poor Mercury and Saturn, my two personal faves, are often at risk of getting cancelled by angsty guests. But I still adore them and their feisty, crashy dominance.

Yet I personally have no time for a Venus gong. In fact anything to do with an A note, the fundamental tuning of that particular planet, gives me the ick. That note, and the accompanying frequency of the Venusian gong, stirs up unsettled discomfort for me, and whenever I'm subjected to its gritty lullaby I always have the rebellious urge to grab the mallet out of the player's hand and hurl it out of the nearest window.

I don't think that's anything to do with Venus as a planet or concept, or the innocent player on the receiving end of my inner wrath. But what I DO think the planetary gongs help us to wrap our brains around is that we are all tuned uniquely. One person's delicious, sensual frequency of dreams can be coffin nails on a blackboard to their neighbour. It's important to remember that sound healing is neither linear nor consistent – with such an array of frequencies firing through your human vessel, not all are going to be smooth landings.

A fair few are simply going to crash.

Back to the gongs. Why am I giving so much airtime to an instrument which above all the others you are probably the least likely to hand over your dollar for?

It's a fair question. I personally think that gongs are among the most powerful and immediate of the sound healing orchestra. Their polarising tendencies can really help us to remember that not everything is for everyone, that our own unique composition gives us an authentic self – physically, emotionally, mentally and energetically – one that is unlike any other cellular structure on the planet. The frequencies we need to find our autonomous state of self-healing are perfectly individual to us.

That's the message of the gong. Embody your own frequency. Just do you.

"Music sets up a certain vibration which unquestionably results in a physical reaction. Eventually the proper vibration for every person will be found and utilised."

George Gershwin, composer and pianist

It was a whole 15 years later that I finally had the opportunity to play the very same giant golden gong that I had found in East London, this time at a gathering in a marquee in the beautiful valleys of West Wales, hosted by its owner, who by now I knew to be one of the most pre-eminent sound healers and makers in the business. Standing behind the giant disk as he danced with his pride and joy, his hand-crafted mallets and wands weaving their unique magic across its glittering surface, I felt its vibration searing into my body like shards of silk, and flashed back to that East London venue all those years before. It was one of the most profound experiences of my life. I can still feel the single salty tear rolling down my cheek and the sharp intake of breath as the sound revealed a sacred truth to me, reflecting it back to me from the shadows, illuminating the hopes and dreams of my much younger self.

Sound healing is all about that emotional memory. In that precious experience, I could reach into the Rolodex of my mind and touch every emotion that had been running through me back in the moment of that first encounter.

It's how I imagined the final cinematic vision at the pearly gates – life flashing before your eyes. I could see it all, and feel it all, all it once. It was as if the sound was bringing all versions of me to the surface at once.

What was my truth?

That remains between me and the sound. You'll have to go seek out that magical gong – or another – and ask it for your own story.

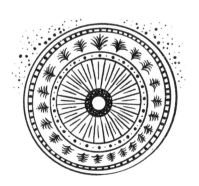

A Splash in the Gong Bath

> Mesmerised by the gongs? Me too. They are relatively easy to record compared to some sound healing instruments, and while you can't get the vibratory effects of the gong online, you can absolutely have an incredible meditative, and often visionary, sound journey experience. They are a hugely effective way of working with binaural beats too, as their natural entrainment is a brilliant conductor for Theta and Delta state brainwaves.

> You can explore a playlist of gong sounds here.

I Want One of Those

> Wind gongs – smaller, flatter gongs that suit hand-held play, are a great entry point for self-sound-healing.

> 30 or 40cm (12 to 15¾in) diameter is easy to handle and ideal for self-practice or working with a partner at home.

> Choose a couple of different mallets to accompany your gong – one instrument can sound like ten different ones when you use different tools!

Playing Tips

› Stand up – playing is a full body action. Brace the weight of the gong with your shoulder but move through the hips and torso. Try moving to the sounds and notice your physical motion entraining to the ebb and flow of the sound.

› Use a harder mallet for rhythmic heartbeats. Strike close to the centre of the gong and let the sound fade almost fully before the next strike.

› Use a softer mallet (wool or sheepskin head) to gently and repeatedly tap the gong closer to its edge, creating a shimmery wall of sound.

› Introduce motion and experiment with how the sound travels when you swing the gong or swoosh it side to side.

› Working with your partner or pet, practice sweeping the gong around the body, and playing it above each chakra point (see Chapter 9, The Wheels of Life) in turn. Just be careful to avoid clattering it near their ears – always strike it at a distance and then bring closer to the body once the vibration is active.

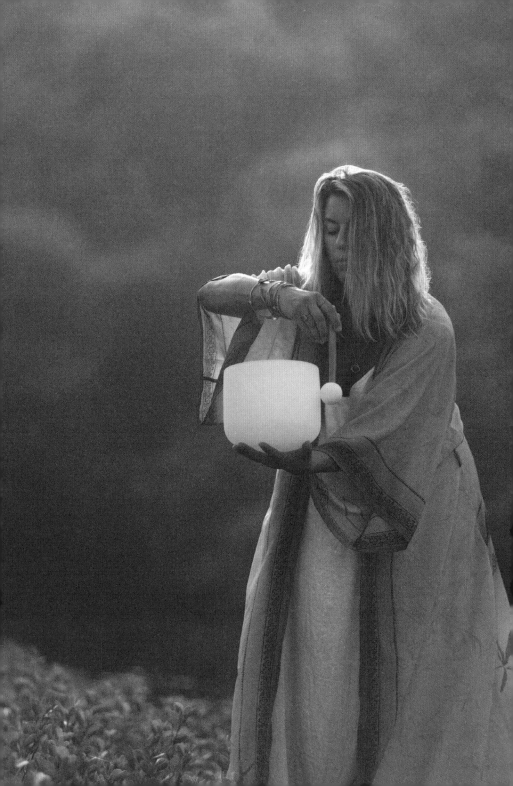

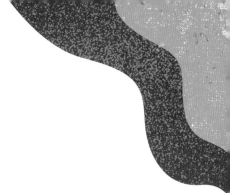

CHAPTER 6

The Sound of Earth and Fire

" *If you want to find the secrets of the universe, think in terms of energy, frequency and vibration.* " Nikola Tesla, inventor and electrical engineer

Suddenly, it seems that singing bowls are absolutely EVERYWHERE.

I'm guessing it's probably one of the reasons you're here. It feels as though every yoga studio in the West is heaving with crystal bowls and soft-focus adverts offering relaxation, deep rest and (my personal trigger word of the century) nourishment. But why the hell not? Crystal bowls do integrate beautifully into so many sacred spaces and healing practices, and it's magical that so many folk, once erring on the side of suspicion of these crystalline crucibles, are now being gently called to receive their ultra-accessible benefits.

While gongs are steeped in some kind of visceral rock music royalty and many of the other sound healing accoutrements have a gently hemp-and-hippies vibe that still sends the masses reaching for the exit button, singing bowls seem the polar opposite of intimidating, and feel completely aligned with the modern wellbeing movement. Easy on the eye, readily available and perhaps a shade on the Kardashian (read: populist) side of sound healing.

But that would be to do these gems a monumental disservice.

And equally gut-punching would be anything other than a stellar write-up for the notably less glamorous but divinely profound metal bowls – usually called either Tibetan or Himalayan as whether hammered into being in India, Nepal or Tibet, their provenance is nearly universally of the foothills of those majestic mountains. They too hold the richest narratives and healing power, forged from and within the roots of the earth.

So let's learn about the crystal bowls phenomenon – and their slightly less sexy but equally potent cousins, the metal singing bowl.

Singing bowls create sound on the simplest of principles: friction. A wand or mallet is gently wafted, dragged or rubbed around the edge of the bowl, and the resulting vibration that begins as gentle hum in your bones gradually grows into a seismic roar, which when played with control and care never fails to blow the minds and hearts of anyone in the near vicinity.

It's a primordial sonic boom, and one of my very favourite sounds.

What's the difference between crystal and metal singing bowls – apart from rather a hefty wad of cash and the need drive with a lot more consideration when transporting your precious passengers?

Much like the wider concepts of sound healing and sound therapy, the two main types of bowl are opposite and somehow equal. Crystal singing bowls evoke pure tones that speak of celestial energy, light codes, the future, space and somehow a deeply feminine, Shakti energy.

Himalayan bowls are generally much lower in pitch (I use the term generally and in the truest sense of the word – of course there are higher pitched metal bowls as there are lower pitched crystal ones) and have always felt to me as though they connect

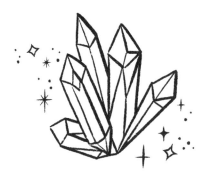

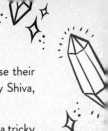

inherently to earth, to ground, ancestry, history and legacy. Perhaps because their lower pitch mirrors the lower octave of the male voice, they feel inherently Shiva, or masculine.

Singing bowls are a wonderful way into self-healing with sound. They CAN be a tricky learning curve in terms of coaxing that sacred song out of them, but I do have to tell you, that never changes! I have some bowls which are incredibly vocal and sing with ease and grace at the slightest touch. Some are shouters, in a 'last orders at the bar' kind of way that can have me gritting my teeth when they get too outrageous in a soundspace. Some literally will NOT give up a note, no matter how much you stroke them, reassure them and learn their every nuance.

They are unique cellular beings, as are we. Their individuality is part of the magic.

METAL MAGIC – THE ANCIENT SOUND OF EARTH

Traditionally, metal bowls are said to have been made of an alloy of seven metals representing the planets, the chakras... the power of seven is an alluring theme but I'm not sure that all great singing bowls truly hold this composition. Actually, the best ones I've played are a brilliant bronze alloy (copper, tin, and a splash of zinc), like gongs. But I do like the idea of trace metals making up the magic seven – and depending on your own persuasion and practice it may serve you to think, feel and experience sound in these terms. Maybe don't lick your bowls though, just in case they DO contain lead!

Metal bowls have an incredible resonance when struck directly, and offer a richly harmonic baritone when rubbed around the edge – it's fairly difficult to write about singing bowls without finding yourself tangled in euphemism but let's leave it at the fact that gently rubbing a wand around the edge of a bowl can create the most magical tonality.

The harmonics of the metal bowls really lend themselves to binaural work, and are excellent meditation tools as they draw the mind into a state of deep relaxation and focus at a surprisingly supersonic pace. They are a simple and powerful addition to your self-sound-healing practice, and I encourage you to explore them with an open heart. Some more ideas on choosing metal bowls follow...

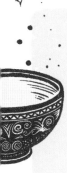

A Mini Masterclass: Choosing Metal Bowls

> Always look for hand hammered bowls if you intend to use them for healing. The machine made or decorative ones (often carved with attractive mantra or Hindu symbolism) are pretty, but do not have the same resonance and sound quality. Test them out and you'll hear the difference!

> About 12-20cm (4¾-8in) diameter is a nice starting point for your first bowl.

> If you plan to play a few bowls together, download a tuning app and check the note of each bowl by striking it with the heel of your hand and holding your the microphone end of your phone inside the bowl without touching it. If the meter is bouncing around a lot, it's not such a clear tuning. A steady note indicates it has been well tuned!

> Consider the octave and pitch of a bowl if you intend to use it to accompany a chant or mantra, as the human voice is mostly pitched in octaves one to four (one being a very low male voice and four a higher female voice). Many smaller metal bowls are octave five or higher, making them pretty shrill and difficult to overtone along to. Use a tuning app to check yours before you buy – the octave is the small number after the note. For example C3 will be lovely to chant to for most people. F5 will be more like a high doorbell!

> Experiment with different mallets and wands, as each will create a very different sound and sustain on your bowl. Think about the size of your bowl when choosing tools – a huge mallet will be muffled on a smaller bowl, while a small wand will not get much out of a giant bowl. If you have a chance to test a few before you buy, do.

> Strike the outside of the bowl about an inch below the rim and explore for the 'sweet spot' – unique to every bowl, where the sound is the truest. You can mark the spot with a marker pen to help you find it consistently until your muscle and sonic memory kick in!

Playing Your Metal Bowl

Three ways to work with just one metal bowl:

1. KUNDALINI ACTIVATION

Sitting down, hold your bowl in front of your torso in your non dominant hand, and gently rub the wand around the outside rim in slow circles. Once the sound has developed, waft the bowl down towards your pelvis and then up the centre line of you body to your forehead. Repeat until the sound fades, and then repeat the process two more times.

2. HEART OPENER

Lying down, place your bowl on your breastbone over the centre of the heart space. Use the middle finger of your non-dominant hand to stabilise the bowl, being careful not to touch the inside of it with anything other than the very tip of your finger. Use a harder mallet to strike the sweet spot and feel the vibrations ripple downwards into your body. Let them fully fade before repeating twice more.

3. MORNING MEDITATION

Seated, hold your bowl in your non-dominant hand. Begin to bring the sound up by rubbing the wand around the outside rim as you inhale to the count of four. Lightly tap the rim of the bowl once, creating a strong bell-like sound as you hold your breath for four. As you begin your exhale through the lips, use the wand to pick up the vibration around the edge of the bowl and gently draw it out to the count of eight. You can tap again at the bottom if you like, to mark the switch from exhale or inhale, or just continue with the wand straight back up to the top of your inhale. Repeat for as long as you like – about ten minutes is a perfect morning meditation.

FUSED IN FIRE: CRYSTAL BOWLS

Crystal bowls are generally made of 99.992% quartz. Remember the teeny tiny crystal fragments in the Swiss quartz watch, all the way back in chapter one?

It's that, but EXTRA.

The clue is in the name with crystal bowls – they embody the earth frequency of quartz, but the alchemical, futuristic energy of the 5D senses, the ones we touched on in our Theta brainwave journey. They have a trance-like, spacey quality that tends to knock even the most determined pragmatist into a slightly trippy state of mind.

They are significantly easier to play than metal ones and that's a fact (trust me). They are also the most magical way to embrace chords, octaves, and the musicality of sound healing, as they hold such pure tones, almost angelic in quality, and it's very easy to hear notes dance with each other and ascertain what sounds glorious and what feels distinctly crunchy on the ears and nervous system.

Whereas metal bowls are individually handmade (the sound-worthy ones, at least) in a fusion of earth, fire and (hu)man, crystal bowls are pretty universal in their birthing process, and it's one that I get asked about endlessly.

Just HOW are these cosmic creatures created?

It's alarmingly simple. Quartz silica sand is poured into a bowl shaped mould, and fired at blistering 2200°C. The resulting bowl is infused with the transformative power of that furnace, and the high vibration amplification qualities of the source material. The high – almost total – crystal content is what gives crystal bowls their energetic qualities and in my opinion, speaks to a higher frequency of consciousness.

Because the moulds are consistent and controllable in a way that a guy bashing a bit of metal in an open flame is not, crystal bowls are always spot on for tuning, which is defined based on the mathematics of the mould – every note has a different mould and you'll notice if you see a set of bowls together that their rims all have different depths.

And finally....

Be mindful of overplaying! You can end up knocking yourself into quite the zombie state if you spend extended periods on your bowls, so be gentle as you learn.

Species of Crystal Bowl

CLASSIC FROSTED
Usually white but sometimes dyed in rainbow colours
to represent the New Age chakra system.

The sturdiest, heaviest and loudest crystal bowls – due
to the large soundwave forms they create..

FROSTED FUSION
Similar to classic frosted but with selected gemstones or precious metals added to the
quartz silica – most commonly amethyst, rose quartz, emerald, gold or platinum.

ALCHEMY BOWLS
Premium bowls which are overlaid or fused with additional gemstones
and minerals. Quieter in volume but more resonant and purer tone.

SUPERGRADE™
Advanced alchemy technology, these are 100% crystal (all other
bowls have a trace <1% of other minerals) and usually overlaid
with the most premium gems and precious metals.

PRACTITIONER BOWLS
Have crystal handles, so they can be played while moving. Often a
slightly purer tone as the bowl is not resting on any surface at all so the
vibration is truly undisturbed. Suited to professional use only.

Playing Clinic: Getting Your Bowls Grooving

Whatever bowl you have in front of you, there are some universal truths:

1. Be patient – let the sound rise slowly

2. Speed is your volume button when using a wand on the rim.

3. The patterns you make on the bowl are your tone of voice – experiment!

4. Be gentle when striking – always aim for an inch below the rim and start very gently.

5. It's a full body movement – when seated, move your hips and core to the rhythm.

6. Feel and intuit – don't feel compelled to make continuous sound. Silence is a noise too.

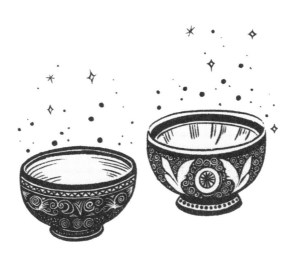

A NOTE ON CHORDS

As we discovered in the last chapter, you don't need to be a musical genius to get stuck into sound healing.

But when it comes to singing bowls in particular, it really does help to have a basic grip on intervals and chords. Otherwise, for all the intuitive play in the world, you'll just be bashing away making random sounds, which will sometimes sound great, but very often not. When notes land in a discordant mess, the spell of sound healing can be broken while the human ear tries to unravel the sound it's being subjected to!

I'm often asked if you need a full set of singing bowls to play them, and the answer of course is NO. You can benefit from the healing power of sound with a single bowl. But if you were looking to invest in a couple of bowls to build a little more depth and reach in your sound healing journey, my advice is always to buy a set that can be played as a chord. You'll simply get much more mileage out of them. Arm yourself with a tuning app when you choose metal bowls, and for any type of bowl use the table here to check the most readily available chords, and read the following section, The Language of Musical Intervals, for more explanation.

BASE NOTE	PERFECT 5TH
C	G
D	A
E	B
F	C
G	D
A	E
B	F#

TRIAD CHORD	NOTE
C Major	C – E – G
D Major	D – F#– A
F Major	F – A – C
G Major	G – B – D
A Major	A – C# – E

The Language of Musical Intervals

OCTAVE – A frequency of double or half the base note. In words of (almost) one syllable: same note, different pitch. Octaves give a sense of space and expansion. For example, if you have a larger C bowl and a smaller C bowl, they share an identical note but one will sound higher than the other (clue: smaller bowl, higher pitch).

FIFTH – The combination of a base note and the one that sits 5 full steps above it. Sometimes called the Perfect Fifth, and said to be the basis of pretty much ALL musical history. If you only have two bowls, make them a 5th apart.

CHORD – A combination of three or more notes/pitches played simultaneously. When played harmonically, this sounds lush. When one note doesn't sit tidily in the team, you'll crinkle your nose. For three bowls try to choose a yummy TRIAD chord that feels good in your unique body.

Don't forget that you can practice chords on a piano, guitar or any other instrument you have to hand. You'll soon find which ones resonate for YOUR body – creating that sense of home that sends juicy shimmers down the spine and warmth into the heart – versus the ones that are your personal purgatory. Like poor old A Major is for me. Give me a D Major all day long!

Singing bowls offer a beautiful bridge between the healing power of sound and a whole library of healing modalities, intersecting elegantly with reiki, yoga, therapeutic touch, counselling, tarot and crystal healing, just for starters. If you're looking for an accessible way to introduce sound healing into your life and practices, these bold, beautiful bowls whether metal, crystal or a symphony of both, are your ticket to ride.

A final note:

While it's not especially hard to get a sound out of a singing bowl, it does take practice and yes, training to get your skills and knowledge to level that is safe for sharing with others. It's important to note that working physically on any body other than your own with bowls really should be left to a professional.

BUT that doesn't mean you can't explore the power of sound through the bowls on yourself, and on your willing friends and family in your private space! That's what this book is ALL ABOUT. Go have fun!

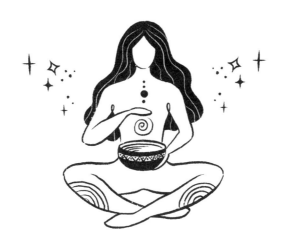

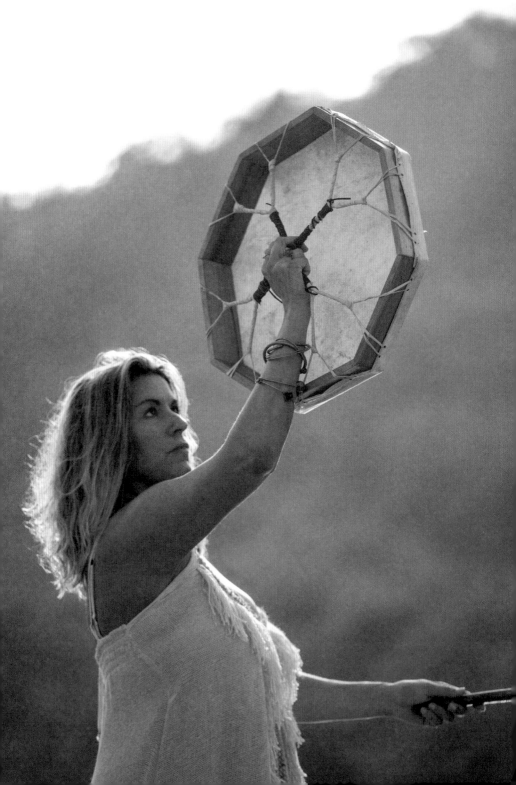

CHAPTER 7

The World is Sound

"When we have learned techniques for harmonic toning, the human voice is able to create nearly every frequency, at least within the bandwidth of audible frequency."

Jonathan Goldman, author and musician (Healing Sounds)

After that odyssey through crystal chords, binaural bowls, and 1970s rock documentary, let's take a beat and roll all the way back down the hallways of ancient history.

Because although we now have an incredible scientific understanding of how vibration affects our bodies and brains, it's easy to forget that sound healing is nothing new. Humanity had sound WAY before we had language, and the first peoples didn't need quantum mechanics and complex neurobiology to understand the incredible healing and powerful properties of the sonic landscape.

They just knew.

Among the first to know were the Aborigine communities of what's now northern Australia. Clocking in at a possible 40,000 year history, one of the earliest instruments we have record of is called a yidaki. It's still in use today, although you might be more familiar with its descendant, the didgeridoo. The early First Nations people are said to have worked with this mystical 'dreamweaving' instrument to induce lucid states in which they created powerful rock paintings, while contemporary Aborigine clans have shared that the hypnotic sound of the yidaki is primarily seen as the people's tool for communicating with spirit, bringing them closer to their ancestors and gods.

Let's bend time and journey back to the 26th Century BCE, to another civilisation that was an early adopter of sound healing. An explosion of construction in the 'Old Kingdom' of Egypt saw a string of 22 or so giant structures supposedly based on the mathematical ratio 4:3:2:0 (stay tuned, that matters) thrown up in a hurry along the western banks of the Nile. These chambers universally had channels running beneath them which contained water.

Remember your bathtub experiment?

The presence of water tunnels altered the harmonic state, the frequency of the pyramids, turning them into resonant forcefields. An accident? Well various reports suggest that these majestic structures were at least in part designed as sound healing temples, complete with quartz crystal tables for receiving healing therapies. The Egyptian name for the Bent Pyramid at Dashur actually translates from their ancient language as 'two harmonies'. Oddly enough it has two chambers, with distinctly different frequencies. Perhaps it's another signal through the tunnels of time that the Ancient Egyptians were way ahead of the game.

There are more than enough conspiracy theories and interpretations of the archaeological story of these lands, so without adding to this already rammed library, I'll just mention that I've discovered more than a few theories by people who've dedicated their lives to the study of Ancient Egypt, suggesting that the Band of Peace (an array of 22 pyramids) was designed as a pilgrimage through sound chambers designed to correlate with organs of the body.

Maybe it's just an attractive story for a sound healing afficionado, but I love it!

However, what seems objectively clear is that advanced Egyptian technology, especially around mathematics and astrology, placed sound at the very centre of their universe. It's also consistent with the learnings derived from their traditions that were later picked up by Ancient Greece and Rome, proven mathematically by Pythagoras, and woven into the foundations of modern medicine by Hippocrates.

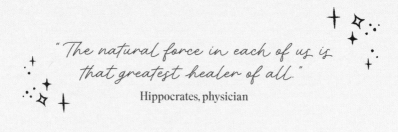

"The natural force in each of us is that greatest healer of all."
Hippocrates, physician

Regardless of your thoughts on a sonic pyramid pilgrimage (one for the holiday bucket list), there is no doubt that the Egyptians had some snappy chants and hymns in their songbooks. They LOVED the sound of vowels to the point of worshipping them, pioneering the practice of 'toning' – manipulating the voice to unlock the power of chant and mantra as a vibrational therapy. In fact, the Egyptians held the seven vowel sounds of their language so sacred as healing tools that they wouldn't even write them down (or scratch them into a hieroglyph), instead their ritualistic chants have been passed down orally.

The Egyptians were among many of the early civilisations who valued the voice – our first and most potent instrument – as a sound healing tool. Musicologist Laurel Elizabeth Keys writes in her book *Toning: The Creative Power of Voice*, 'Toning is an ancient method of healing. The idea is to simply restore people to their harmonic patterns'.

Nonetheless they did have a few nifty early instruments out back, including the sistrum, often seen in connection with the Egyptian goddess Hathor. The sistrum – a metallic rattle – was said to create altered realities and encourage healing through bringing the body into entrainment with accompanying music during celebrations and ceremonies. It was also rather handily said to help avert the flooding of the Nile!

A sistrum is a lovely basis for creating your own rattle from natures' gifts. Have a look at the ideas in Rattle & Hum below to create your own.

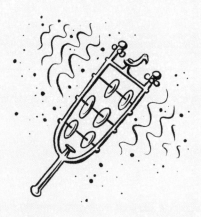

Rattle & Hum

A sistrum, passed from the Egyptians down to the Roman Empire and beyond, is pretty much the earliest percussion instrument seen in western music. You can mindfully craft you own simply by taking a walk in nature.

WHAT YOU'LL NEED TO FORAGE:

› A Y-shaped twig, as strong as you can find
› A handful of acorns, conkers, or any kind of nut

WHAT YOU'LL NEED IN YOUR TOOLBOX:

› Thin picture wire or even strong nylon cord
› Something to bore holes no bigger than 2mm ($^1/_{16}$in) diameter

HOW TO MAKE IT

Make a hole in each of your found treasures and thread some of them onto a length of wire or cord. The foraged nuts should be able to slide freely back and forth. Tie the wire/cord between the forks of the twig, making sure it is stretched tight. Repeat the process to make a second row. The sistrum should make a pleasing swooshing sound when waved from side to side.

You could also make a sistrum using bottle tops, metal discs or crystal beads, whatever speaks to you.

If the twig is big enough, you could carve your own symbols or mantra into the handle, or decorate with feathers, beads or colourful cord.

Make it your own.

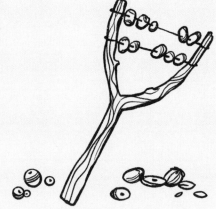

THE UNIVERSAL INSTRUMENT –
AWAKENING THE VOICE

Can you remember where you first connected with singing, the voice, chanting?

Perhaps some of the memories you explored in the earlier chapters of this book revealed lullabies in a childhood bedroom, or singing along to family favourites in the car. Don't forget that chanting is a powerful tool in football stadiums, pop concerts, and protests, not to mention nearly all religions.

For me, and I reckon for more people than you might expect, some of my earliest sonic memories were formed in church. Whether you were a regular Sunday-schooler or never got closer to the cloth than a televised royal wedding, the likelihood is you'll have encountered some version of chant and hymn inside those echo-laden walls. Or at least on the terraces or streets of your childhood.

I was raised a Catholic, and was sent to a secular school. For me, the fragrance of rich frankincense and myrrh is forever connected to the church we used to go to every Sunday, and to my memories of sitting tucked out of sight in the odd little cubbyhole along the side aisle, clutching my flute and faffing about with the hymn sheet. Mr Spark, our friendly school music teacher, would play the church organ, and a motley crew of us ten- and eleven-year-olds would play along, occasionally in time and generally not. My favourite part was always the call and response chants. They felt quite dreamy and everyone seemed to be able to stay in tune for those.

Which is unsurprising, because their roots were in the Gregorian chants of the 10th century, when the early Christian monks crafted trance-like chants using a six-note system called hexachords.

Like the Egyptians, the Greeks, Romans, Tibetan monks of the Himalayas, monastic peoples of Southeast Asia, the ancient Chinese, the First Nations from Siberia to Peru to Ethiopia and pretty much ALL folk before them, the Christians had realised that chanting had an unmissable and tangible influence on human physiology and mental wellbeing.

These Gregorian scales (by the way, they were named for Pope Gregory I, in case you were wondering) evolved the concept of unaccompanied plainchant – which is exactly what it says on the tin – during the Middle Ages, and formed the basis of the modern musical notation.

Scientists have concluded what anyone who has hung out in ashrams or monasteries for more than a minute can affirm – monastic singers are incredibly peaceful, breathe very slowly, and need very little sleep. In fact, contemporary studies have shown that those who regularly chant register lower heart rates and blood pressure numbers during their vocal exercises than at any other time of day.

Suddenly, a morning shower chant sounds like a REALLY good thing, doesn't it?

Of course, chanting doesn't have to be religious AT ALL. I'm using the Gregorian example from my own experience and because it links to perhaps nature's greatest mathematical magic – solfeggio frequencies – which we'll get to. But meanwhile, we can take chant and put it together with overtoning, the early Egyptian iteration of chant which you could define as making sounds without words.

› Try it now – say 'AH' as if you were in the dentists' chair, and then start making shapes with your lips while keeping the sound going.

› Now try again and don't move your lips but see if you can move your vocal cords and tongue around to change the sound from INSIDE your mouth.

› Next, see what pours forth when you make shapes AND try some vocal gymnastics.

Fun, right?! It feels a little odd at first, but overtoning actually IS the most natural thing in the world.

Finding Your Voice

Here's some easy ways to bring chanting or overtoning into your day:

MORNING SHOWER – There's no better place to let loose, and we already know your bathroom has the best acoustics! Set your voice loose with some freestyle overtoning and notice your mood shift by the time you reach for the towel.

YOGA OR MOVEMENT – Whether you're starting the day with sun salutations or a run, try soundtracking yourself with Gregorian or Vedic chants in your ears. It will be strange at first, but you'll be surprised at how your breath changes.

MEDITATION – Try a seated meditation with your spine nice and tall and shoulders back. Lift your chin ever so slightly – an open chest and throat really helps a good chant to break free. Try a simple eternal OM:

› Take a BIG inhale and really pour the breath down the back of your throat until you feel your chest lift and fill. Take a couple of more or these to awaken your lungs fully.

› At the top of your inhale, begin your OM. Technically, it's pronounced o-w-m (and spelled Aum). Try not to move your lips too much. Let the sound move from deep inside you and flow out with your exhale. Keep the exhale SLOW and imagine the chant carrying the breath out, rather than the breath pushing the sound. It will make sense in action!

› Play with extending the owwwwww- and shifting the shape of the word to -wwwwmmmmm halfway through your exhale.

› As soon as you run out of breath begin your inhale, trying not to rush but filling your lungs again in one clean sweep.

› Belt out another OM. Keep going. Try setting an alarm for three minutes and build up to ten over a few days or weeks of practice. You'll be amazed at the change in your lung capacity as well as the anxiety-blasting lowered heart rate to start the day.

NADA BRAHMA & THE YOGA OF SOUND

As we're on subject with the amazing tool of chanting, it would be remiss not to take a quick drive-by of the Vedic tradition, the practitioners of which have also long been aware of the wins around using specific sounds and mantras, not just for healing but for creating vibrationary resonance in the body and in physical spaces of all kinds.

The entire Hindu tradition (and thus the entire global yoga obsession) is based upon the Vedas – essentially a collection of chants, mantras and hymns, written in the beautiful Sanskrit language sometime around 1500-1200BCE, when the Egyptians were handing over the reins of sound healing in the New Kingdom to the embryonic Greek civilisation.

The Vedas describe the creation of the world as having emerged from sound – the primordial cosmic sound of OM. My very favourite phrase from this rich cultural milestone is NADA BRAHMA.

It means THE WORLD IS SOUND.

Consequently the phrase NADA YOGA is the term used for the yoga of sound; creating yoga (union) with voice, chant and vibrations in the body. It's why your friendly local yoga teacher invites you to activate your practice with sound, and where the beautiful practice of kirtan, or devotional song, has its far-reaching roots.

Vedic mantra is such a powerful tool for healing, not just because of the sonic benefits of receiving chanted words into the body, but also because of its affirmative energy. If you haven't tried chanting to remove obstacles from your day – give it a go. You won't be disappointed by the endlessly healing combination of sound, harmony and hope. We'll take a deeper look at mantra and the sounds of the chakras in the next chapter.

"Starting with DNA, the whole body unfolds into many levels and at each one... the sequence of sound comes first. Therefore, putting a primordial sound back into the body is like reminding it what station it should be tuned to."

Dr Deepak Chopra, author and Professor of public health at University of California, San Diego

The Power of Drumming

While we're in storytelling mode, let's take a final sweep past some other fascinating traditions and cultures who have gifted us sound healing legacies. The shamanic drum is often associated specifically with the First Nations of North America, and especially the Great Plains, so it might be a surprise to hear that it actually originates from the Siberian tundra, from where it worked its way across the American Arctic.

But shamanism – loosely defined as the quasi-religious practice of communicating with the spirit world via altered states of consciousness – covers boundless practices and peoples. Historians generally agree that shamanism predates pretty much all organised religion, and stretches back well into the Stone Age, suggesting that indigenous peoples from east Africa to Peru to the Arctic Inuit had identified the benefits and powers of working with a potent beat and its visceral energy long before anyone had even considered what a musical note might be.

The drum is variously believed to be a channel for connecting to spirit realms, a trance tool, a sonic sage stick for banishing the bad vibes; and a practical healing medicine – an excellent method of pushing blockages and negative energy out of the body.

It is also an excellent vehicle for brainwave technology, effectively shifting our conscious state through the deployment of a rhythmic vibration that entrains the brain, and eventually the body.

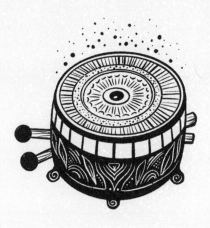

I especially love how the heart and the bones seems to respond so viscerally to the drum in my sessions, with guests often reporting a primal sense of connection to earth and nature as the beat moves them into a Theta brainwave.

Drumming is also a great example of how vibration and sound healing works with extra va-va-voom in collective and community environments. In indigenous and shamanic cultures across all timelines of civilisation, the drum was used to bring people together – connecting them in a shared rhythm. Sometimes huge drums needed a whole community to play them, or perhaps manufacture was a group project.

If you need any more evidence of the power of drumming, just take a look at how often it is used to create and keep rhythm where crowds gather; unifying energy and connection between people from protest picket lines to the carnivals of Notting Hill or Rio, and the hand-drumming of gospel choirs. One of my favourite examples of potent collective drumming action didn't use any instruments at all – the synchronised rhythmic clapping Queen's performance of *We Will Rock You* at Wembley Stadium (London) remains one of the 20th century's most spine-tingling live music moments, and in the many gigs I've seen at that famous venue, I don't think I've been to one that hasn't tried to emulate the potency of that accidental yet totally natural magic.

You can probably see why I spent so long talking about entrainment now... it's the absolute soul of sound healing.

From ancient painted wooden drums to skinned frame creations and the African djembe, drumming sits at the very heart of human transformational ritual. While there are of course many complex drum patterns, and invocations that accompany them to induce particular supra-conscious states or call on specific deities or spirits, ANYONE can feel that drumming is really a very simple conversation between hand, heart and brain.

Just start tapping the nearest hard surface to you now, whether tabletop, edge of the bath or steering wheel. See how quickly you fall into a sonic pattern?

As well as the many iterations of the drum, shamanic culture has also introduced a whole host of sound tools to humanity, not least one of my favourite categories: the rattle.

Rattles are not just the domain of the nursery, in fact they are used alongside the drum to assist in disrupting blockages that arise when the body's vibrations have fallen into disharmony. In shamanic tradition, they would also be used to draw out and dismiss dark spirits and energies that had surfaced through the drumming.

Rattles are a SUPER EASY way to connect with sound. In the healing sense they can be shaken over areas of the body that feel blocked or unsettled. It may sound counterintuitive, but try it and be very surprised as you notice areas of tension begin to disperse under the targeted sound.

Also worth a mention: the reason rattles are such comfort blankets for babies is that they encourage sensory stimulation and focusing on just one sound – Alpha brainwaves, right? – which helps little ones out of anxious emotions.

The same principles applies at all ages. Try using a rattle softly but continuously to create a lush elemental sound that can help move your brain out of active overwhelm and into a less overwrought sate. I also find they are great for rerouting an ADHD or distraction-riddled mind back to topic – speaking from a LOT of experience. I keep a cute little wooden rattle from Bali on my desk and go to it like a stress ball.

Percussion is the lingua franca of sound healing – the universality of its rhythmic language transcends time, place and skillset.

And it's so simple. All you have to do is pick it up and PLAY.

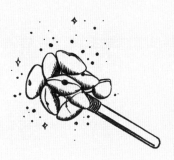

Kitchen Cupboard Rattles

Rainsticks and ocean drums are types of rattles that create sounds that tune you into the water element. They are beautiful emotional soothers and help both kids and adults with auditory processing, visual motor skills, and impulse control.

WHAT YOU'LL NEED:

> A small cardboard box.

> For a rainstick shape, something like a bottle box is great, or for an ocean drum, try a small shoebox or cereal carton.

> A collection of grains and pulses – about two cups for a rainstick, three or four for a small ocean drum.

> Smaller grains like couscous or rice have a softer and quieter sound than larger ones like lentils or chickpeas. A mixture of different types creates a more oceanic sound!

> A parchment bag or roll of baking paper.

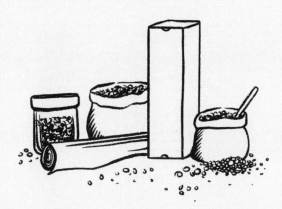

HOW TO MAKE IT

› To make a parchment/baking paper bag, cut a rectangle of paper the same height as your box and of a length that equals the widths of all four sides of the box when added together. Tape the ends of the paper together to make a tube, then tape the bottom edge. Your parchment/baking paper will make an inner bag that needs to fit reasonably snugly inside your container. Use scissors and tape to get it just right.

› Fill your bag with a mix of large and small grains – I like lentils and rice!

› Seal your bag with tape and fit it inside your cardboard container. Ideally, secure the bag to the cardboard on all four sides (easier in a flat box, if you are working with a bottle box you may want to deconstruct it first and then rebuild it around the sealed paper bag).

› Close and seal your box... you're done!

› Now you can gently tip your DIY ocean drum from side to side or turn your rainstick up and down. Go slowly and enjoy the wave-like sound of the grains rattling across the baking paper.

TIP: for a more durable option, check out your local garden centre for materials – hollowed bamboo or eucalyptus stems are a good starting point.

You could also paint your rattle or tie feathers, crystals or anything else talismanic to it. In the communities of Africa, Indonesia, India and the Americas where rattles crafted from nature are currency, you find the pulses housed in something like a coconut shell, or carved wood, sealed with colourful fabric or skin wraps.

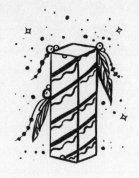

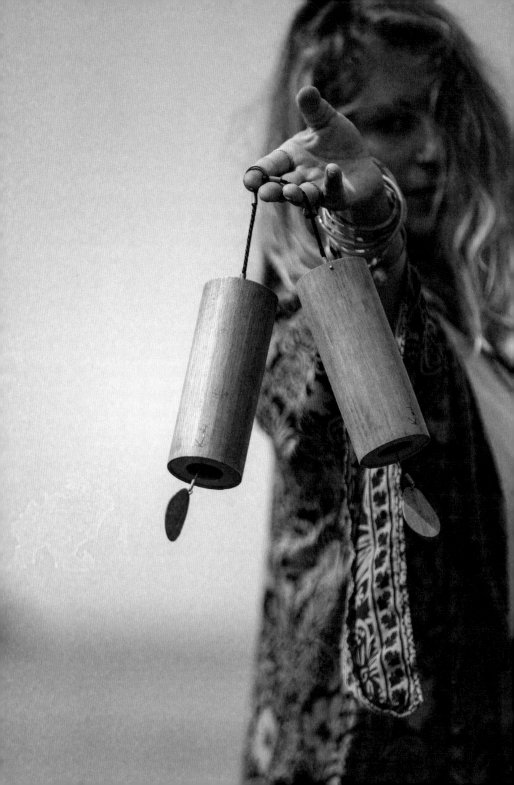

CHAPTER 8

Modern Life is Rubbish

" Music can minister to minds diseased, pluck from the memory a rooted sorrow, raze out the written troubles of the brain, and with its sweet oblivious antidote, cleanse the full bosom of all perilous stuff that weighs upon the heart." William Shakespeare

Are you stressed out?

I know I am. Overwhelm. Responsibilities. Emotional fatigue. Too much to do. Too many phones. Wearing expectation and external demands like a chunky ball and chain. What even is time and how can I get more of it?

You know the hollow feeling when you repeat a word so much it completely loses all meaning and just becomes a noise? I feel that way about the word stress. The word has become so synonymous with modern life it often feels like an omnipresent overcoat for the human experience, rather than its all too tangible reality: a chronic and potentially fatal condition of the psyche.

And body of course. Because we certainly do know that the body keeps the score.

Britpop legends Blur certainly made a catchy point with the record from which this chapter borrows its title. Their observational musical summary of the state of society perfectly epitomises the ubiquitous struggle. Because if not entirely rubbish, then modern life is certainly inherently stressful. Humanity, at least in the developed world, seems hellbent on eating itself alive in a perfect storm of overwork, financial crisis, porous personal boundaries, digital exhaustion, expectation, fear and perennial emotional meltdown.

In fact it's a reasonable assumption that one of the reasons you have this book in your hands right now is that the long reach of the mental health epidemic has touched you or your people in some way – and you know that sound healing has the potential to ease you through life's labyrinth of stresses and strains.

You're right – it does. I feel that it has the power to be one of our most impactful resources in the fight to bring humanity back from the brink of a collective nervous breakdown.

Let's get stuck in.

The Space Between the Beat

Neurologist and ayurvedic doctor Kulreet Chaudhary MD shines a spotlight on the intersection of conventional and vibrational medicine in her excellent book, *Sound Medicine*. She underlines the entrainment between heart and brain as the very cornerstone of our mental health, and one that is directly accessible via sound.

Put simply – if your heart is in pain, sadness and fear, and entrains those emotions to your brain, you'll start to THINK those low-vibe feels too.

It works in both directions. If the brain is transmitting positive codes it can entrain the same to the heart. If the heart is radiating with all the euphoria of an unexpected day off in a heatwave, the brain gets on board and attunes to that same inner dopamine.

Let's check the top-line science, because it really does matter when it comes to the impact of sound on our nervous system.

We know that the heart is in the paid-up service of our autonomic nervous system, the regulatory kingpin that flicks between the sympathetic and parasympathetic subsystems.

The rhythm of the heart, the HRV (heart rate variability), is your own inherent beat and, contrary to popular belief, it's not consistent or should it be confused with the overall speed at which your heart beats. We're talking about its capacity for responsiveness..

Try this analogy on: your HRV is a drummer.

A world-class drummer (hey, Dave Grohl) sets the pace for the rest of the band, but is also able to be flexible. If the lead singer suddenly has an ego moment and changes the set list halfway through the show, a great drummer will simply keep things funky, adjust the tempo, and without missing a beat, get the band back on track.

Just like one of those stumbling-over-your-own-shoes accidents you style out as if it was intentional.

However if the drummer is insistent on sticking to the scored rhythm despite everyone else going rogue, it's all going to descend into a speaker-crunching mess pretty fast, with everyone playing out of time.

This rhythmic disorder is what happens to our HRV when it's not in coherence – by which I mean, not able to be attuned, flexible and responsive to the different experiences your body is moving through in every breath of life.

When we get stressed out, frustrated or lost in the red mist our fight-or-flight sympathetic nervous system hikes our heart rate and tells the brain to pack its bags for the anxiety train. First stop – shallow breathing. Then, it's a one way express straight to fear, panic, lack of focus, irritability and at the end of the line burnout, breakdown, or cardiac arrest.

Obviously, there's a lot more complexity in the neurotransmitters that do the heavy lifting in the brain, but you get the idea.

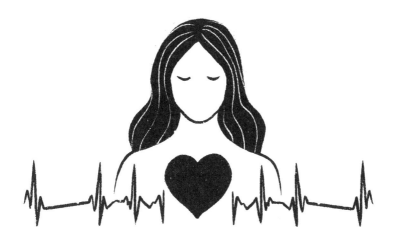

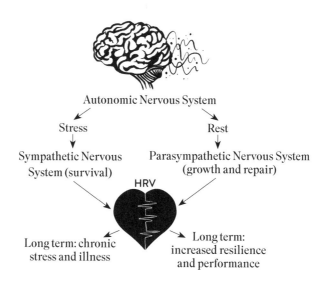

Autonomic Nervous System

Stress   Rest

Sympathetic Nervous   Parasympathetic Nervous System
System (survival)   (growth and repair)

HRV

Long term: chronic   Long term:
stress and illness   increased resilience
                               and performance

However in the soundspace, it's the rest-and-release parasympathetic system that is activated by the frequencies flooding the body and brain. This kickstarts a much slower train, meandering gently through reduced heart rate, regulated breathing and a long cool drink of calm at the oasis of... well how does peace, love and light sound?

Yes it's a cliché, but oh-so-appealing when you think of the murky alternative.

With the sound regulating our nervous system back into balance, the heart and mind can resonate and entrain to a coherent rhythm, giving us a nice high HRV. This greater capacity for responsiveness equips us to cope with the curveballs and chaos of life.

Which seems a lot better than just popping a pill to tell the brain to misread its own signals, don't you think?

Try it Out

> It's tricky to check your HRV without equipment and an app, but you can get the idea by carrying out a standard pulse and breath test to observe the differences in your system functions before and after listening to a sound bath recording. The 4-4-8 pattern breathwork you've learned in chapter two is also a useful tool for regulating HRV.

YOUR NATURAL SONIC BIOFIELD

While we are dancing with the real-life experience of a joyfully regulated nervous system, it's a good moment to mention the biofield.

Perhaps you know it as an aura, kosha, or energy shield.

It's another one of those inconveniently invisible parts of us that doesn't show up on conventional scans.

But you know it's there.

And because we now have machines that can reliably measure the vibrations of the field around the brain and heart (EEG and EKG machines) – science knows it's there too. Or at least, it's being grudgingly persuaded by mounting evidence.

This forcefield of electromagnetic frequency is something that aligns with the philosophies and teachings of many ancient cultures, and is the trigger for a plethora of well known (and oft-appropriated) smudging or sacred cleansing rituals which were designed to keep this field cleared of debris, disharmony and general energetic grub.

As we know, drumming rituals also were used across the ancient world and continue to be woven into contemporary sound baths in order to shift the vibration of the human biofield.

Slaloming from science back to spirit for a moment, let's discover how the ancients had already worked out what the heck the biofield was, centuries before the Force was a twinkle in Obi Wan Kenobi's eye....

The Vedic texts (the source material of Hinduism, and thus yoga, dated to roughly 1200BC) teach that the body is made up of five layers or skins, called koshas. The koshas radiate out from our most dense layer – our physical body.

As we journey outwards through them and beyond the edges of our 'skin-suit' we get close to our spiritual core, embodied in the fifth and final layer of our being. This layer – let's call it the Bliss Body to keep things simple – is exactly what it sounds like. Spiritually speaking, it's where we can touch enlightenment, nirvana, pure light, divinity.

In terms of physics and the quantum field, the outer koshas are said to be where we can connect with our universality at a cellular level, touching the constellation of consciousness.

In practice? Through the natural laws of resonance, not to mention a whole bunch of pretty cool molecular interactions, sound baths allow us to spend time deeply connected to our outer layers of being. In the parts beyond the edges. In the extratingly part of our own electromagnetic field, which is in constant interaction with the rest of the cosmos, time, energy.

Call them koshas, biofields, whatever you need to to get clear on the fact that YOU take up a lot more space than you thought. And that space is made up of vibration. Sound. A lot of the theory around the these cosmic aspects of our being suggests that western medicine has become obsessed with the first layer – the physical body, and that's why humanity has got stuck on the starting blocks when it comes to connecting to our purpose, and to each other.

It's a theory I really like. Not least because when carried to its natural conclusion, it becomes obvious that introducing sound healing, amongst other modalities such as reiki, acupuncture etc, is the tonic that will grant us access to the rest of our own biofield, and in the end, our TRUE POWER.

When that happens, surely our ability to heal, to find balance, to experience the glorious extremes of life's glittering potential, will be realised. Nirvana indeed.

The koshas are imperceptible to our conscious senses but rendered very much present once we are immersed in the cosmic waves of a sound healing space. After blissing out in a dreamy sound journey, many people report the sensation of feeling their body extend way further than the mirror shows it.

Practice the You are the Forcefield exercise that follows to tap into your own energetic biofield. What do you discover?

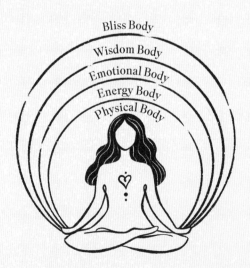

You are the Forcefield

Test the concept of the koshas by coming into a quiet, meditative state and holding your hands in front of your chest, the palms 1cm (½in) or so apart.

As you focus on the space between your palms, can you begin to feel it vibrate and light up?

Allow your hands to move apart and choose one to glide up your forearms and across your body – slowly and mindfully, don't touch, just sense what is going on in the space immediately off your physical form. Play around with moving your hand further away from your body and then closer in again.

If you have tuning forks or a singing bowl you can also use that to 'comb' the area around 1-20cm (½-8in) off your body.

What do you discover?

Don't worry if nothing obvious comes up at first. Tuning in takes time and you may want to try this again after a sound bath to see what feels different.

Get Forked

Now that we know about the biofield, and how keeping it clear and balanced is fundamental to our wellbeing, let's get right into one of the most practical and immediate sound healing tools out there. Because if there is a silver bullet in the sound healing world, this is it.

They provide instant gratification (yes, really), they require zero musical skill, and they're really accessibly priced.

Too good to be true? Say hello to TUNING FORKS.

I generally play with a pretty extensive array of instruments in my signature soundscape sessions – giant gongs, crystal bowls with uplighting, amazing rare black metal bowls from the Himalayas, antique flutes, a whole fleet of drums, a guitar, decks. Yet the question that I get asked almost more than any other at the end of a session is about the very last whisper of vibration guests receive – usually the most gentle, almost imperceptible touch of a tuning fork to the third eye.

All that insanely expensive equipment that takes me hours to load in and set up, and the thing they ALL want more of is a tuning fork! It's a good thing I have a sense of humour.

Generally stainless steel or preferably, pure grade aluminium, tuning forks look pretty innocuous and to most people like something they dimly recall from the nurse's office at school, or from a childhood doctors dress-up bag. Certainly not exactly cutting edge sound healing technology.

And yet, that's exactly what they are.

Tuning forks are almost ludicrous in their simplicity – just strike them against something resistant (see The Daily Tune Up) to create a vibration, and then direct it where it's needed.

That vibration – which you will be able to hear as a pure tone sound – can either be passed through the biofield (now you know!) or in the case of weighted forks, can be applied directly to the body to send the frequency medicine direct to source.

Of course, there are many years of certified technical trainings available and indeed required in order to safely practice on other people. Amongst other things you'll need a decent grip on anatomy, to understand acupressure points, and be properly trained in therapeutic touch.

Plus, there's an awful lot of frequencies out there to wrap those brainwaves around. But for self-care, you'll be blown away by what a daily dose of self-administered fork can do for you.

I've mentioned that we all have our own overall frequency – between 5-10Hz is usual for the human body – and within that our organs each have their own individual frequency too. Many practitioners subscribe to the idea that organs vibrating out of their natural frequency is a manifestation of disharmony, and is where disease comes from.

The simple maths – and this goes all the way back to Hippocrates and the healing chambers of Ancient Greece, teaches that returning the organs to their preferred frequency creates natural balance, resonance and wellness. Deepak Chopra agrees.

> *"The body is held together by sound;
> the presence of disease indicates that
> some sounds have gone out of tune."*
>
> Deepak Chopra

With an eye (and ear) on the therapeutic space, tuning forks give us the resource to actively target conditions and symptoms with a high degree of specificity, harnessing the power of sound to directly approach issues that cause us pain and problems.

We know for example that 128Hz is a particularly useful frequency for targeting joint and muscular pain, and that 50Hz usually elicits an almost immediate sense of calm and peace (it is said to offer a direct line to the sympathetic nervous system). 68Hz is a brilliant meditation aid especially when used on the brow bone (energetically, the third eye chakra), and a combination of 256Hz (C) and 384Hz (G) creates the classic peachy perfect fifth that invites the two hemispheres of the brain into resonance.

I work with tuning forks directly on the body to deliver these frequencies, and this is an accessible, easy method that you can try too. Tuning forks are super accessibly priced and a great way to begin your journey with sound healing. These are my top tips for getting started with them:

THE DAILY TUNE UP

I've been doing this sonic cleanse-tone-moisturise for years. It's like morning stretches, but for your vibrations!

› Breathe naturally, and very gently slow your breath down just a touch from its resting rate.

› Tap the fork lightly against a rubber ball or your kneecap to get it vibrating. Always hold the fork around the stem – if you hold the fork part itself you'll halt the vibration.

› Once vibrating use your wrist action to direct the stem of a weighted fork towards the body and gently touch down – no pressure required – to the desired spot.

› Remember the golden rule: weighted forks are on body; unweighted are to be wafted through the biofield without making skin contact.

Three is the Magic Number

Here are my favourite three quick-wins for tuning fork practice:

BREATHE – use a weighted 50Hz fork at the higher heart chakra – an inch or so below where your collarbones meet. Instant anti-anxiety meds. Where do you feel the vibration?

DREAM – use a weighted 68Hz or unweighted 432Hz at your third eye chakra, between your eyebrows, for a cosmic boost and shortcut to creating what you really want in life. Notice what comes to the front of your mind as the vibration sinks into your skin.

BALANCE – Using C and G perfect fifth unweighted forks, hold one in each hand and breeze by your ears. Cross your wrists in front of your face, switching the forks to sound in the opposite ears. Play with moving them around in figure of eight shapes. You'll probably notice one ear or one note dominates. Notice for how long, and if that dominance fades.

Stick to around three repetitions of each practice. Any more is vibrational overkill! The tuning forks are brilliant for assisting the body in releasing more nitric oxide, which supports elevated cellular function. This scientifically proven process happens quickly and imperceptibly, so just a short tune-up is perfect.

Think of it as like a sonic gua-sha massage: less pressure = greater impact.

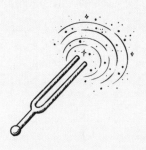

Musical Mathematics

If you go digging around for tuning forks, it won't take long before you stumble over something called the SOLFEGGIO system.

Remember the Gregorian monks and their hexachord chants? The scale used to craft these power hymns is called the solfeggio scale, and contains six special frequencies which as early as the 10th century had been identified as having a particularly profound impact on the body and mind.

Yes, it may sound right on the edge of calculus nerd territory, but the six solfeggio frequencies sport some pretty sexy maths (yes, really). They can all be reduced to either 3, 6 or 9. Nobody knows exactly where they originated, but that man Pythagoras had a bit of a thing for these particular numbers too – they form the basis of his famous triangle – simply look at the degrees in each corner. Incidentally it was he who first nailed the practice of reducing numbers, a cornerstone of both numerology and sacred geometry.

Which in turn, weaves seamless macramé magic with sound healing.

"There is geometry in the humming of the strings
there is music in the spacing of the spheres."

Pythagoras

Is there really such a thing as co-incidence? Were the Catholic monks of the Middle Ages receiving divine transmissions about the healing power of certain sounds, or were they just particularly nifty with the abacus?

Either way, the strange case of the solfeggio frequencies remained buried in history until around 1900, when engineer and inventor Nikola Tesla (yes, the plug-in cars are named after him) developed new work exploring the connections between music, vibration, electricity and a few very specific numbers.

Like Pythagoras some 1500 years earlier, Tesla knew he had discovered something special about the numbers 3, 6 and 9. Taking the Greek mathematician's calculus to the next degree, Tesla looked at the magic numbers as sounds and frequency, applying this sacred numerology to his many inventions.

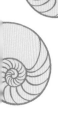

Nobody is quite sure of the history around what happened next, but when much of Tesla's research vanished after his death the story of the solfeggio frequencies seemed to fade back into obscurity... until 1970 when one Dr Joseph Puleo rediscovered them while researching numerical patterning in the book of Numbers, part of the world's most famous book – the Bible.

Healing frequencies had been hiding in plain sight for 1000 years.

Why am I telling you this meandering story about numerology?

Well, the early research into the DNA-based impact of solfeggio frequencies has shown that they are attached to particular healing outcomes.

And the super fast way to access these frequencies and direct them into the body?

TUNING FORKS.

Increasingly, instrument makers are also offering singing bowls in these frequencies too, and my favourite little tongue drum is the way I bring them into my group healing sessions.

So do these magical, mythical frequencies actually WORK?

There is still a long way to go in terms of evidence-based research, but with almost the whole of modern western music derived from the construction of these six key frequencies, I think it's certainly worth taking a deeper look around for the fire that has created 1100 years of sonic smoke.

As always, I think the best way to decide is to be your own experiment. Try them out, and YOU decide if the monks were onto something.

I think they were.

Physics teaches us of the innate connection between life, space, mathematics, matter and music. Nature's sacred geometry is what creates beauty and resonance in the natural world – which we can observe translated into our very bodies.

Have you ever noticed the similarity between our lungs and the structure of trees?

Between sea shells and the architecture of our inner ears?

Nature's harmony relies on geometry, mathematics, pure form. We've known for thousands of years that music is mathematics dancing off the page.

This is the very foundation of the healing power of sound. Frequencies that restore harmony.

What do YOU think?

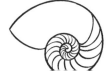

The Solfeggio Six

If Vedic practices and yoga are your groove, you may like to align these frequencies to the chakras too, as a method of helping to drive awareness and intention of their different energetics.

396 Hz — Releases fear and negativity (root chakra)

417 Hz — Facilitates change and evolution (sacral chakra)

528 Hz — DNA repair and self confidence (solar plexus chakra)

639 Hz — Heals relationships and harmonises (heart chakra)

741 Hz — Supports self-expression (throat chakra)

852 Hz — Awakens intuition, offers a bridge to higher self (third eye chakra)

Post 1990s, an additional three frequencies were added (using the same magic maths favoured by Pythagoras, Tesla etc) and modern sound healing and vibrational medicine recognises these tones as harmonious accents to the original six.

174 Hz – Pain relief and biofield cleanser

285 Hz – Rejuvenates tissues and organs

963 Hz – Activates psychic and supra conscious channels (crown chakra)

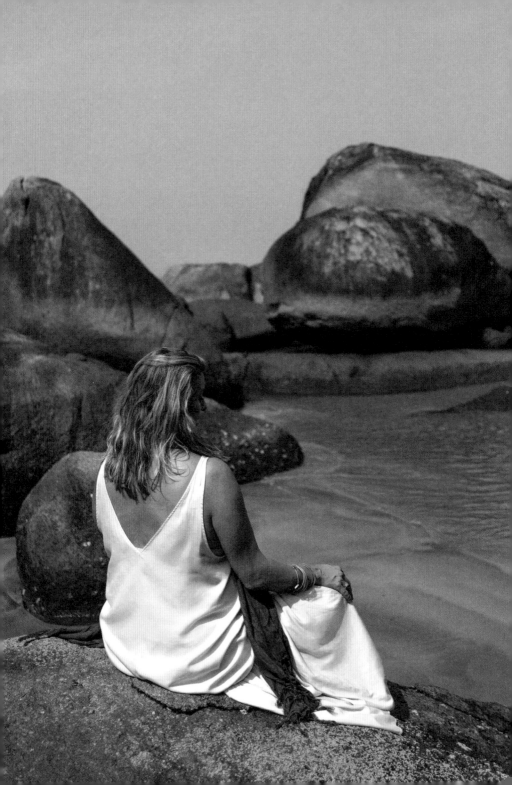

CHAPTER 9

Expanding Consciousness

"The experience of life in a finite, limited body is specifically for the purpose of discovering and manifesting supernatural existence." Pythagoras

So far we've looked at a hefty chunk of the science around sound healing. Landing this feels crucial to a modern reading of soundwork, as despite the zeitgeist vibes around all things sound, it's still all too easy for it to be misunderstood as the territory of fake gurus and silver bullets.

But it's also a good moment to re-assert my own personal mantra, that sound healing sits across the intersection of science and spirituality. They co-exist, interact and harmonise beautifully – one aspect cannot be without the other. Both parts are needed to weave the song, to make the melody. Together they make up a super special sauce for self-healing.

So let's put down the textbooks and jump aboard the technicoloured, surround sound, spiritual train. Because on the other side of the science is a fascinating myriad of mind-bending, consciousness-expanding experiences, just waiting to be unlocked and explored.

The Magic Carpet Ride

A sound bath – like the ones I like prefer to name 'sound journeys' or 'soundscapes' – is loosely defined as an experience where sounds are projected into and around the body for healing benefit. You may see a sound bath promoted as sound meditation, immersion, or perhaps a good old fashioned gong bath. Either way, you can be fairly sure that the intention is broadly to create a field of resonance that invokes major and mesmeric change. Wrapped up of course in whatever unique gifts, storytelling and integrated rituals each individual practitioner offers.

My own gift wrapping usually features accessible astrology, psychedelia and plant ceremony, with the odd sprinkling of crystal healing, and a finishing glow of reiki. I think that providing as many entrance portals as possible for people to find their way into the soundspace can only be a good thing.

While some sound folk remain purely focused on the relaxing, soothing benefits of sound – and doubtless there are many – I'm personally most ignited and inspired by the potential for tangible healing, as well as transcendence while in the soundspace.

What do I mean?

When I talk about transcendence, I'm simply asking you to step into the world beyond your physical realm. To transcend the edges of your physical being. To expand into the domain of the right brain – a place of vivid imagery, rich emotional imagination; a hotline to intuition, to higher consciousness.

When you transcend the body, you speak to the soul.

The spiritual side of sound healing travels the corridors of the mind that we simply can't reach in the day-to-day of our productivity-fuelled lives, which are usually too busy trying to get the food shop done and stay on top of the social media tsunami to consider the realms of hyperconsciousness.

The game-changer is the fact that pure-tone sounds delivered to the brain flick the right hemisphere ON, plugging us straight into our psychic selves (yes, you DO have a psychic self – we just happen to live in a western, capitalised world where it's not valued or understood, so you've probably switched it off for survival).

Suddenly our sensory perception dials up a few gears, and we can see beyond the limitations of our functional senses.

We can really SEE, with our whole being.

In practice, this means that the sounds may hold space for you to experience visions, see faces known or unknown to you from this realm or another; hear an internal dialogue, experience touch or physical sensations on your body, and witness the very fabric of life through new and unseen lenses.

Remember that moment in the film *The Matrix* when Neo first sees the threads of binary code that make up reality beneath the simulation?

It's just like that. This is the place where spirituality gets its iridescent wings on and sweeps us away from our physical existence.

When I'm in full flow, illustrating this experience in my opening chat, this is often the moment when I look around the room and catch a few saucer-like eyes. I say to those people and to you: take a deep breath.

You are perfectly safe in the soundspace cocoon.

In fact there are very few contraindications that would exclude anyone with any medical issues from sound healing – and when experienced online or purely through the voice, there are even fewer, as the visceral vibrationary aspect is out of the mix. However if you're feeling anxious about the 5D experience, and the word psychedelic has you visualising the shadier bits of the 1970s, fear not.

To defuse the fear, simply return to the power of INTENTION. Craft your own journey through setting your course mentally and emotionally before the soundship departs. The frequencies will always move towards blockages first, and if the one you arrive with is fear or shaky nerves, the sound waves will simply speak to your anxiety, soothing you into a chilled parasympathetic state and guiding you into a gently regenerative groove.

The power is always within you to choose exactly what shape your sound experience is destined for.

So where do you want to go?

The Wheels of Life

When its comes to unravelling the connections between our spiritual selves and sound, the Vedic culture set an early bar. The chakra system, with which any western yogi worth their eco-mat will be familiar, is directly derived from Vedic teachings, although versions of the theory show up in a huge variety of cultures, religions and wisdom traditions from Kabbalistic ritual to Zen Buddhism via Christianity, Sufi mysticism and more.

Whichever theological container resonates for you, the takeaway is that the chakras are the energetic organs of our subtle energy body, invisible on an x-ray but very much tangible in the soundspace and all spiritual practices.

Each chakra is a kind of cosmic computer, correlated to an element and with its own energetic purpose in bringing balance to our soul's journey. The basic tenet is that each 'wheel' (the Sanskrit translation of chakra, or technically cakra) must 'open' in linear order from root to crown in order that our life force energy may rise to its potential.

Depending on your affinity with tantra, acupuncture, Japanology or Chinese medicine you may know the concept of life force as kundalini, prana, chi or ki. Regardless of provenance, the principle remains that this vital life force directly links our physical health to our spiritual wellbeing.

Back to the rising kundalini. Nature's divine order dictates that once each chakra is vibrating in harmony, the serpentine spiral of rising energy can connect ALL the chakras, exploding at the highest point (the crown) in an orgasmic firework said to gift spiritual peace, unconditional love and enlightenment.

It's a kind of supra-conscious geometric crystal maze, ending in nirvana.

The vibe, not the band.

In order for the chakras to provide the channel for this expanding consciousness, they individually need to arrive in harmonious symphony. The practice of yoga asana (the making of the shapes on a mat) in order to prepare ourselves physically for meditation, is part of this process.

But we can also arrive at this theological hedonism through sound, because each chakra has its very own vibration. By chanting or invoking these sacred sounds, we can activate each of these wheels of fortune, one by one, releasing ourselves into a spiritual awakening.

So what are these mystical, primordial sounds that offer the magic button to spiritual bliss?

Well what they are NOT is anything to do with the concept of musical notes being associated with specific chakras. In fact, this much vaunted connection is in no way rooted in any of the spiritual texts or traditions from which humanity tuned into the energy body – it's actually part of the New Age rainbow revolution of the 1970s.

In fact, similarly to the ritual soundwork of Ancient Egypt, the early sound healing practitioners of the Indian subcontinent held melodic overtoning and harmonious chanting in the highest esteem. Their musical adventures extended beyond single words to sequential ragas and mantra, whole passages of sound with complex inbuilt healing frequencies. These were said to be delivered at very specific times of day, season or for certain ailments or energetic malfunctions or desires.

These pioneers of sound healing knew that working with spiritual awakening via the chakra system wasn't just about creating a singular sound or vibration in the body; they knew that the whole shebang needed a hell of a good 'WHY?'.

It had to be about intention.

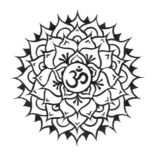

That's a huge part of why I always cue a guest's intention as we begin our sound odyssey. I'm there to drive us through the soundscape. But it's the guest's own intention that steers, that sets the course for their experience.

Coming back to the concept that links chakras and musical notes (as I KNOW some of you in the back are still itching to ask...), I think that the whole extravaganza simply remains an enduring and alluring myth. However, although I take on the concept with the appropriately large pinch of salt, it isn't without some beneficial threads.

We've been trained by society to seek order and structure amidst the capitalist chaos, and the seven-note system offers a familiar, easeful portal. It's a way in.

As a result, I often open my sound baths with a chakra meditation and I do find that the organisation of notes alongside chakras can provide really helpful clarity for our overloaded, over-processed brains, and reminds guests of the actual presence of their energy body.

So while the easy alignment of western notes to a system which we know to be infinitely more musically, energetically and spiritually complex then seven convenient chakras does rather smack of simplification in pursuit of a quick sell, it does at least give us a tangible melodic journey from one chakra to the next. Which has its value.

Much like our journey with the gong, the idea of single tones landing in very specific parts of the body – physical or energetic – can also really help us understand that we are each receptive to different notes and tunings.

For example, I feel that my D bowl, associated with the sacral chakra in the western gaze, really DOES stir things up in that area for me. But conversely my C bowl, supposedly aligned with the root chakra, actually always resonates in my solar plexus. So I just use them in the way that resonates for me.

It will be different for you. Each energetic organ, just like each physical organ, vibrates with its own unique frequency. Your sonic fingerprint is completely yours.

If a note resonates for you and feels juicy and alive and energising in a particular area of your unique structure, then that's yours to own.

A great way to work with the chakras individually is to use the bija mantras, or 'seed' sounds that were identified in the earliest texts of nada yoga – the yoga of sound. Rather than a randomly allocated musical note, these ancient Sanskrit sounds are designed to be chanted using the power of the voice to create vibration inside the body – both physical and energetic.

Of course if you want to use your singing bowls alongside them, with the 'correct' tunings or not, that's your prerogative. I do, because I just like how it all sounds together. It's a cute way to weave the old and the new; bringing together the primordial sounds of our energy body with our tangible physical voice and the man-made tools of the trade.

Use the Toning the Chakras exercise at the end of this chapter to get connected to your chakras through sound.

The following is an illustrative guide to the chakras and their correlations, with added western musical notes. As always, take what serves you, and feel free to leave the rest.

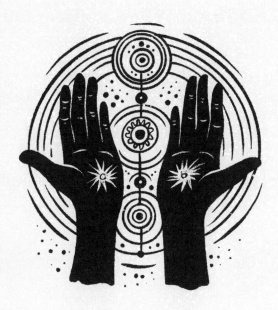

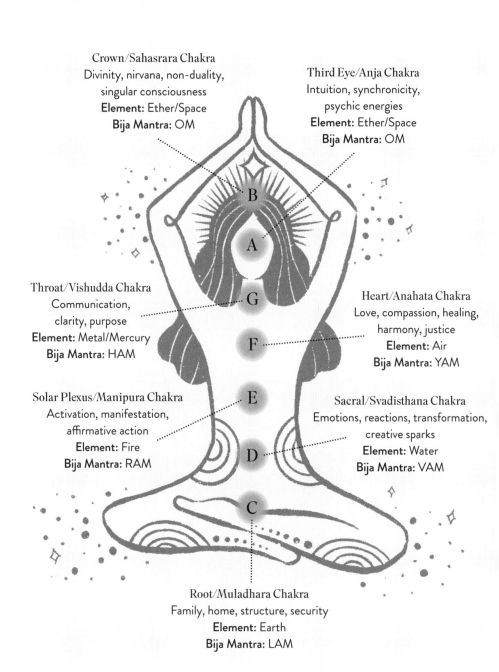

Crown/Sahasrara Chakra
Divinity, nirvana, non-duality,
singular consciousness
Element: Ether/Space
Bija Mantra: OM

Third Eye/Anja Chakra
Intuition, synchronicity,
psychic energies
Element: Ether/Space
Bija Mantra: OM

Throat/Vishudda Chakra
Communication,
clarity, purpose
Element: Metal/Mercury
Bija Mantra: HAM

Heart/Anahata Chakra
Love, compassion, healing,
harmony, justice
Element: Air
Bija Mantra: YAM

Solar Plexus/Manipura Chakra
Activation, manifestation,
affirmative action
Element: Fire
Bija Mantra: RAM

Sacral/Svadisthana Chakra
Emotions, reactions, transformation,
creative sparks
Element: Water
Bija Mantra: VAM

Root/Muladhara Chakra
Family, home, structure, security
Element: Earth
Bija Mantra: LAM

SO, EXACTLY WHAT WILL YOU FEEL IN A SOUND BATH?

Experiencing sound in your chakra system is a great starting point for your more spiritual sound journey, and as it can fully unplug your mind from the physical body, is also a supersonic way to relax and de-stress.

I often describe it as the magic carpet, a journey that reminds me of the fantasy adventures of childhood mixed up with every futuristic film I've ever seen, all painted up in a dazzling array of colours and finished with a strobe light. It's like a festival in your mind.

But we all know that even the greatest festivals have those shadowy stages in the far corners of the field, the ones with unfamiliar acts and possibly no bar, that seem a long walk back to your tent.

In the soundspace, guests sometimes notice a heaviness or blockage in their throat area, where the chakra that supports our communication systems is found. In a world stuck in a perpetual loop of digital overdose, it's unsurprising that many sound travellers notice that this chakra is where balance and energetic clearing is most immediately needed.

The sensation can be surreal at first, a little magic roundabout and not always entirely pleasing. But as the sound and vibration weaves its magical way through the chakra, the healing often manifests as physical release in the form of coughing, which softens as the sounds finish and the chakra begins to rebalance.

Another common experience is the sense of crushing pressure across the heart chakra, often a symptom of anxiety and fear.

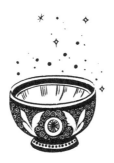

Yes, I agree, having a flashlight over this sort of vibe doesn't exactly sound like something you want to part with your hard earned cash for.

The good news is that the experience of the sound bath is all about infusing this energetic centre with lightness and harmonious peace as it dissolves the stress frequencies and gets your heart chakra feeling all lovely, light and free again. Yummy.

Headlines? It's not unusual to notice the sound targeting a particular chakra area while in a sound journey. By cross referencing the relevant themes in the preceding chakra diagram, you may notice exactly what and where is showing up for healing for you – sometimes the sound can be truly diagnostic and help us get to grips with something we've been burying, or can encourage us to look at something we've been dodging on the to-do list.

Be reassured that whatever gripes or pains you're bringing to the space whether physical, emotional or spiritual will be given a very good rinse and wring out by the sound. It can be a washing machine.

But you'll be nice and clean afterwards.

I've recorded my classic chakra-awakening sound journey for you to experience, giving you a chance to tune into the energy body and your own higher consciousness realms. I hope it takes you out into the galaxy of time and space, journeying on your very own magic carpet.

In the end, so much of sound healing leans into spiritual intuition – so the only thing that truly matters is the question I love to ask all my clients as they reach for their journals at the end of a session:

HOW DOES IT MAKE YOU FEEL?

Toning the Chakras

A simple mantra based exercise to raise your vibration and self-sound-heal using the instrument everyone can play – your voice.

> If available sit on the floor in an easy cross legged position, or lie down flat on your back.

> Begin with a couple of rounds of 4-4-8 breath (see Chapter 2, What's Your Natural Tuning?).

> Place one hand on top of the other, both palms down; place your hands as low down in front of your root (aim for the pubic bone) as you can, and with eyes closed take a deep inhale through the nose and exhale the sound LAM.

> Keep the sound going until you are totally out of air. Take a very low intentional inhale and repeat twice more.

> Move your hands up to the sacral chakra – a couple of inches below the navel, and repeat with the next mantra: VAM.

> Continue through the solar and heart, and for the throat chakra place one hand on ether side of the neck, bringing the heels of your hands to touch in front of your throat.

> For the third eye, try a prayer mudra (position) for the hands with the thumbs touching the brow bone.

> For the crown, place the heels of the hands softly on the top of your head and keep the palms apart – as if you were literally putting a crown on.

> For a longer practice or as a standalone meditation try repeating the whole cycle three times. If you are a yogi you might like to add the mantras to a sequence of chakra activating postures.

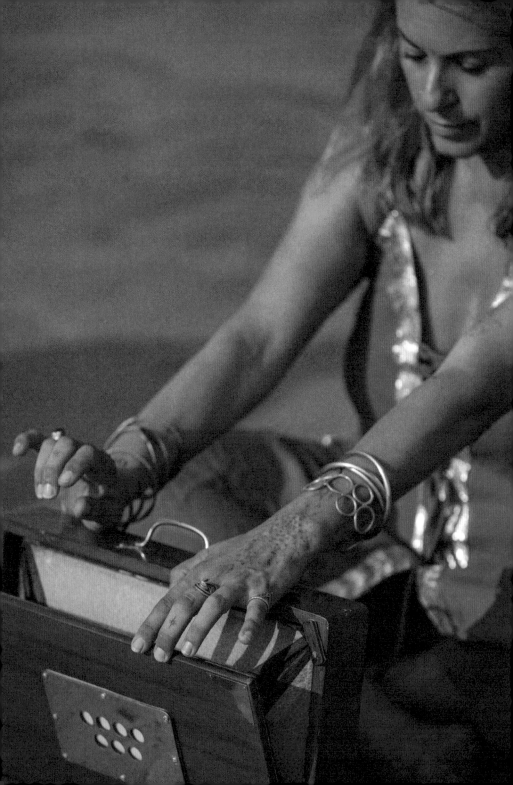

CHAPTER 10

Living a Sonic Life

"What makes us feel drawn to music is that our whole being is music, our mind and body, the nature in which we live, the nature which has made us, all that is beneath and around us, it is all music." Hazrat Inyat Khan

Hopefully by now you've learned that the rich history, powerful science and spiritual wisdom around sound healing combine into a practice that is about so much more than creating a softly-lit, sage-scented healing cocoon.

Tapping back into the knowledge of how sound permeates the body, we know that from a PHYSICAL perspective it can have enormously positive benefits for people living with neurological conditions such as Parkinson's disease, or multiple sclerosis.

We know that the deep connection between music and memory makes sound healing a brilliant resource for those living with dementia, Alzheimer's or other conditions related to cognition and neural processing.

And what we now know with increasing nuggets of mind-blowing research and lived experience is that sound can make a supermassive-black-hole-sized impact on our mental health and emotional wellbeing.

Stress, anxiety, depression and PTSD are amongst the most debilitating conditions that third millennium Earthlings are locked in battle with, and sound is a tool that offers us both tangible physical healing and significant shifts in our emotional landscape.

It can create powerful and significant change at a cellular level, shifting our internal vibrations to alter the way we process emotions and experiences. It's CBT for the nervous system, retraining it to actually evolve into a supercomputer capable of unlearning old ways of coping, rinsing out old trauma, and rewiring programming that is past its sell-by date.

It's a tool that allows you to live the life you deserve, released from the struggles of adapting your brilliant body to the reality of a world it wasn't built for.

There are countless studies that show just what an incredible impact sound and vibration can have on humans, and you can find signposts to these in the appendix if you want to dive into some serious science and feed your thirst for detail. I'd love to get into the bones of that powerful work right here and now, but we'll end up down a very deep rabbit hole indeed...

And really, the takeout that matters is that sound medicine works.

Here's a non-exhaustive list of just some of the benefits that have been explored, researched and observed anecdotally by practitioners and patients alike:

> Lower blood pressure

> Regulated respiratory rate

> Increased immune response

> Boost to our natural opiates such as dopamine

> Reduced anxiety symptoms

> Creation of resonance in the nervous system

> Improved circulation and red blood cell performance

> Improved sleep quality

That's just to start with.

A major name in the crossover medical sound healing world is the late Dr Mitchell Gaynor, a respected oncologist. His pioneering approach to cancer treatments in 1990s New York included prescribing chants and sound meditations alongside working on body with singing bowls. He summarised sound medicine brilliantly:

"Sound enters the healing equation from several directions: it may alter cellular functions through energetic effects; it may entrain biological systems to function more homeostatically; it may calm the mind and therefore the body; or it may have emotional effects which influence neurotransmitters and neuropeptides which in turn help to regulate the immune system – the healer within."

Dr Mitchell Gaynor

Dr Gaynor's words remind us that sound works with our bodies on a multitude of levels.

Right back in the early stages of this book I talked about the differences between healing and therapy in the sound world. There is definitely space between them – but when applied as an elixir for the twin-headed monster-under-the-bed of stress and anxiety, I think the two modalities blend into one supersonic powerhouse of a tool.

Because sound healing spaces do offer therapeutic benefits that directly target the causes of conditions, and likewise, sound therapy can absolutely be experienced while dancing on the cosmic clouds of a deliciously dreamy sound meditation.

Especially when it comes to mental health.

That's why the healing power of sound is my own tool of choice, and one I recommend to all human beings with a whole and confident heart.

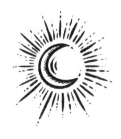

Music of Sound

I've interchanged the words music and sound at various points throughout this book, because I think that they are different sides of the same record. Sound as we know is everywhere and everything, the architecture of the universe. Music is constructed sound; the vehicle by which most of us consciously choose our sonic environment.

"Sound healing differs from music because it purposefully uses the principle of entrainment by directing sound, coupled with intention, to clear physical and energetic blockages, sometimes at the cellular level."

Ashana, musical artist

I like the focus on intention that Ashana leads her definition with. A sound healing space such as the ones she or I hold will offer you a carefully constructed and intentional symphony of therapeutic sound which is of course a great way to experience sound healing in a truly profound and amplified way. I don't for a second want to diminish the value of these amazing spaces and the years of training and expertise on offer!

However, the music you choose to feed your ears with outside of a formal sound healing space can still have incredible effects – and this comes down to being both aware and intentional with the shape of sounds you switch on.

So when you consciously decide what to listen to – when you select a radio station to wake up to, choose the album you are going to soundtrack your drive with, or press play on a track to get you into your running shoes like you mean it – you are making a deliberate and considered decision about how YOU want to feed your brain and body.

This decision holds the potential for sound healing, because it is on PURPOSE. You now have binaural beats, mantra and ragas to add to your playlist library, all of which definitely qualify as sound healing in the classical sense. But you also have the capacity to choose music that makes an impact not just on your ears and your mood, but on your wellbeing. I firmly believe that from Beethoven to Nine Inch Nails; ANY music can be healing – if applied in the right moment and with the right intention.

Shall we go all the way back to page one for a moment?

How Sound Speaks to You

Think about some of your favourite songs. Perhaps after taking this sound healing journey, you might answer the question with a new perspective:

Why do you love them, really?

Is it that never-getting-over-it crush on the singer? Because it reminds you of a version of yourself only available in photographs and memories? Or perhaps it's because the key change before the middle eight sends a shiver down your spine as the particular arrangement of notes talks uniquely to your own cells?

Have you ever felt like someone was singing a song directly to you through the speakers? It's not just about evocative lyrics – your body is attuning to the musicality, the tones, the scales and chords.

Particular voices or octaves just speak to you. This is partly taste of course, and the multiplicity of skills in modern music production. We are certainly in the era of the super-producer, tastemakers adept at tuning into the cultural zeitgeist. But I would argue that if we could get past the part of our musical taste based on cultural coding and tuning into what's big on TikTok, we'd likely find that actually our own taste is defined by our own internal tuning, what our body finds beautiful, at a cellular level.

Some tracks objectively speak to the masses – I mean nobody ever headlined Glastonbury by having an average back catalogue – but perhaps on closer observation you might find that certain keys or types of musical arrangement repeat themselves in a pattern throughout your favourite tracks.

I know that much, as an A major sends me running for the hills, whereas a D minor will always hit the spot for me. Even songs I don't particularly love take on a new texture when I put them into that key. And there's a certain tonality of delivery shared by most of the singers I truly love. Not in every track or all the time, but it's there.

You too have your OWN tuning, your own perfect note and frequency, and you probably haven't even met it yet.

It's kind of like knowing your perfect partner is out there, just over the horizon. And what could be more juicy and alluring than the chance to come face to face with them?

Here's another example of musical magic speaking to the body: the opening line of 'Over the Rainbow' – a song surely nobody needs an introduction to – is objectively evocative because the vocal famously jumps a full octave. We know is a pleasing sound to the human ear because that sonic leap creates a little rush of euphoria, a little hit of dopamine.

Any music that plays around with the perfect fifth is going to create a similar high-powered impact. Interestingly lots of nursery rhymes naturally use this interval, and many of the most memorable theme tunes from cinematic history are built around it.

In fact, we can loop back to Star Wars for the perfect example of a score so expansive that it's impossible to hear the opening passage without feeling the scale and reach of the galaxy, epitomised by stars spiralling into eternity as the opening text scrolls up the screen. That famous melody at the heart of John William's score is built around an opening musical leap of the perfect fifth – pure balance in musical form, a reminder that the eternal battle of light and dark can be won in the geometry of harmony.

The maths of the Force, indeed.

It's so easy to get lost in the universe when writing about sound – but let's come back to your favourite songs, your playlists and your WHY.

As well as the musicality, tonality and entrainment of certain sounds to unique and beautiful YOU – there's the other simple truth that we touched on right at the top of our journey.

Perhaps when you really feel into why you love certain music, it's because the song subconsciously connects you to a time, place, person or feeling.

This is one of the major ways that sound healing through music therapy has become such a significant tool in the important work of supporting certain neurological conditions. A great example that we touched on previously is the case of both dementia and Alzheimer's disease. It's pretty well-documented that music is one of the most connective tools for those living with these degenerative conditions, and classical musical therapy involving singing and choirs is increasingly on the radar of the new breed of social prescribers in modern healthcare.

For the dementia groups I've worked with, although I offer them a group sound healing experience, we're not looking to take those particular guests on a transcendent trip. Instead, the sound journey has truly therapeutic benefits as the frequencies cut past the neurological noise and plug them back into memories and experiences that are dissolving or fading when processed through the conscious mind. Scientists tell us that the precortal part of the brain is activated by music and sounds, and this is the very last part of the brain that degrades when challenged by dementia, meaning that sound memory can still reach someone long after other senses and communication pathways have become blocked or distorted. Experiential work with clients has given me a deeper understanding of how sound work can truly impact chronic conditions, offering a therapeutic solution where conventional medicine sometimes falls short of the elusive answer.

Truly, as the American clairvoyant and enlightenment enthusiast Edgar Cayce famously wrote:

"The medicine of the future will be music and sound."

Of course, the reality is that truly it has always been the medicine of our civilisation, since the first primordial sound rang out across space.

We've just rediscovered it.

It's hard to imagine a reality when we couldn't readily access the entire musical history of civilisation. But now we can almost literally put a cup up to the wall of time, and listen to the chants of Ancient Egypt or our great-grandparents' favourite ditty as easily as we can tune into the latest pop releases. With such a vast library of music available at the swipe of a screen, the scope for greater healing through the power of sound has never been so rich.

Our final journey in sound is into the future.

PLAYLISTS ARE YOUR SUPERPOWER

"Music is the mediator between the life of the senses and the life of the spirit."

Ludwig van Beethoven

As we've dived into ancient and world music traditions and stories, it's obvious that for thousands of years, humans have used music and sound with intention. From the Egyptians to the Eskimos – the ancients knew that while certain sounds undoubtedly had healing benefits and served as conduits for divinity, the biggest sonic boom they left for us was the skill of using sound in accordance with nature's cycles.

From specific ceremonial chants to using particular instruments or songs only after dark, before lunch or on a full moon, these cultures had nailed the concept of living a cyclical life. Their chants, mantras and drumming rituals were the first playlists. And as the world's most accomplished DJs know, what you hear is only half of it.

The rest is timing.

Not just what you listen to, but WHEN you listen, and in what context.

I'm taking a sidebar to illustrate this.

One of my favourite ever live shows that I've been at was the French electronic duo Daft Punk. It was 2006, and I was very much out of my depth at that kind of gig. Sure I loved dancing, and was spending increasing amounts of time in Ibiza. I had managed to pick up that the famous clubs peddled a kind of euphoria not dissimilar to the hazy sunset drumming that took place on nature's dance floor in the north of the island, and I was intrigued. But although the first whispers of sound medicine were running through my veins, it was early days. And I didn't really go to electronic 'gigs' back then. I liked guitars. I had no idea what to expect of it all, but stayed curious. When Daft Punk came onstage they proceeded with a lengthy digital introduction that built a kind of hysterical anticipation that I've never seen replicated, before or since.

The beat was so pulsating, so powerful, the layering of the tracks so artful, the sense of an imminent explosion when the track finally landed was palpable in a lip-licking, barely breathing kind of way. The anticipation was almost excruciating but we all knew

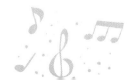

we had to soak up every second of the breathless buildup. It was like watching a long-dormant creature rise from the centre of the earth, unfurling slowly towards the sun.

It was five or six minutes in by the time the beat dropped in what I can only describe as a sonic smackdown and the first track fired into life. The entire crowd seemed to lift off the ground as one. A slow-motion ascension and a collective inhale, and for a split-second I had the idea that the entire festival was suspended in silence. I'll never forget it. It was as if they had woven enlightenment itself into their set.

The timing was so perfect it was almost luminous.

Why am I telling you this?

Because sound is a dance of speed, matter and time. Do you remember the physics?

› Sound is... vibration travelling through matter

› Frequency is... the speed at which the vibrations travel

And the right sound at the wrong time is just a noise.

You know this already, of course. You hear it every day in conversation. On TV. Pitch-perfect comic timing. A sacred pause before bad news. A silent heartbeat before the penalty is struck in a crucial football match.

Timing.

If you've been to live gigs and concerts, maybe you've noticed how important the set list is. The shape of the whole experience lies not just in the songs that are played, but the order in which they land, and the segue between them.

The soundscape is a sum of its parts – musical architecture, performance, intention and timing.

Hold onto your hats – as we're going from 2006's electronic pop fiesta for a final spin round the ancient sound healing heritage of India.

Remember the ragas? These are sequences of musical notes from the Hindu tradition. Neither set melodies nor scales, they are fluid structures which are open to the interpretation of the artist. Technically, the raga is the musical or melodic part of the structure – making up one half of the traditional concept of Indian music. Its non-identical twin is tala. Timing.

These little musical sculptures are designed to evoke specific feelings and emotional responses in the listener, and are specifically designed for different times of day, seasons and to accompany specific festivals. The sound and the timing, together designed for a specific moment, experience or emotion.

You probably have your own equivalent to ragas, buried in your streaming service or smartphone. The core tracks and sounds that make up the backdrop of your life, whether classic favourites that take you back to a decade of bootcut denim and bum bags, or a particular type of production or synth that you didn't even realise was your innate go-to groove.

This is your own form of music therapy – a sonic happy place that brings your energy, emotions and perhaps even physical body into its natural alignment. There are thousands upon thousands of ragas, but musicians who work in the Hindustani tradition might usually work with a repertoire of 50 or so. You may not have a performing repertoire – unless you happen to frequent the local karaoke dive bar or moonlight as a busker on the weekends. But you DO have a listening repertoire to dig into.

So what do you listen to most – and more importantly, why? And learning from my Daft Punk story – how does it all flow together? Does your own personal soundscape evolve seamlessly and continuously, or slalom between genres and timelines in a multifaceted blender?

Both are fine, by the way.

Thankfully, our digital streaming services are packed with helpful tools to help you take inventory of your tunes. What themes can you identify in your listening habits? Use the journalling exercise that follows to help you draw out the stories and make sense of them.

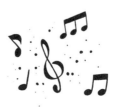

A Sonic Audit

› What's the first thing you listened to every day this week? Is there a pattern? How does it make you feel?

› Do you have an artist/artists/track on permanent rotation (meaning you listen to them every day)? Why? Consider what it brings up for you in familiarity, connection, sense of time/place. Or is it that you just like the music/sound?

› Identify key activities and their soundtracks. What do you listen to when working/driving/exercising? How do your choices support the activity you are doing? Can you identify what exactly it is about your selection that motivates you, focuses you, or distracts you?

› Do you have any 'secret' songs – the ones that are totally leftfield relative to your mainline taste, the ones you are embarrassed to admit to you like (come on – we all have them!)? Can you pinpoint what it is that draws you to the song, despite the cringe factor?

› Do you already have any music or sounds that you see as therapeutic saved in your playlists? How do they make you feel and when do you go to them?

› Do you have sounds for sleeping, meditating or resting? What's the last thing you listen to at night? What does this tell you?

BUILDING YOUR PERSONAL SOUNDSCAPE

By curating your own playlist-driven soundspace you are gifting yourself the power to manage and support your wellbeing, mental health and physical state of being.

Taking your notes from the journalling exercise above, let's build up your own musical universe so that you can use sound with intention and healing even when you're stuck at your desk or trapped in traffic. By the way, this isn't intended to replace your constantly evolving musical taste, simply to help you use awareness to make the most of what you already love, and make space to meet some new sounds that might just be the splash of mojo you're missing. I've also added in a couple of self-sounding practices – feel free to sprinkle these into your day wherever it makes sense to you.

> **Step One:** Identify cycles, patterns and activities. What does your time look like daily, weekly, monthly? Think about when you reach for your headphones or turn the speakers on.

> **Step Two:** How do you want to feel in these moments? Try to commit to just a couple of words.

> **Step Three:** Choose music and sound to bring those feelings into reality – I've given you some ideas to help you get started.

I have wildly different work playlists depending on whether I'm writing (and need to be buried in tunnel vision) or coming up with creative ideas (when I want Theta waves and blue sky potential). This is reflected in the difference between screen time and deep work in the diagram that follows, and you'll probably have your own parallel variations.

You can take these ideas further based on your own natural patterns. I have really different work playlists for when I'm on my monthly cycle, when I notice myself grappling more with concentration as my hormones host their own little disco. It's a great idea to have a little list of your essential tracks to signal key milestones in your physical and emotional week, like a TFI Friday song but for morning coffee, or your midweek team Zoom.

Other cycles and patterns that I recommend playlisting for include the lunar cycles, intention-setting or diarising for the week, and your sacred rest time. But you can use soundtracking as a connective tool for pretty much anything. Just do so intentionally, using the step by step formula above to be crystal clear on what the purpose of the playlist is. If you can bring the music to life with instruments, hand-drumming or even just your voice – you're feeding the connection to the sound.

Intention is everything.

GOAL: Start the day feeling enlivened, activated, awake and alive. ← **MORNING SHOWER/ ROUTINE** → IDEA: Tuning fork activation. Familiar songs you can sing along to help get you into your voice early in the day.

GOAL: Open the voice, release a good hit of vibe-lifting dopamine and plug into uplifted energy. ← **DRIVING OR CYCLING TIME** → IDEA: Connective tracks that take you to positive memories. Strong baseline or percussive beat.

GOAL: A potential trigger so zone out, rest, and take some time in the internal tunnel. ← **COMMUTE/ PUBLIC TRANSPORT** → IDEA: Peaceful tracks that don't fight external noise and keep you in a narrower focus. A time for mantra meditation.

GOAL: Activate fire-starting energy and themes of motivation, manifestation and confidence. ← **GYM/HIIT/ RUNNING** → IDEA: Up-tempo vocals for keeping forward motion. Lots of positive chord intervals. The perfect house music moment!

GOAL: Time for gentle focus. Close down peripheral noise, seek awareness and a more lucid state. ← **YOGA/ UNGUIDED MEDITATION** → IDEA: Repeated chants or gentle vocals lull the mind into a state conducive to flow and harmony. Soft, lilting melodies.

GOAL: Attention, awareness and concentration – for multitasking and alertness without getting overwhelmed. ← **SCREEN TIME** → IDEA: Ragas or mantra chanting are brilliant for keeping you alert and conscious.

GOAL: Develop laser focus, creativity, sparks of genius and a single focus. ← **DEEP WORK** → IDEA: Alpha binaural beats are gold standard. Make sure they are in your headphones for the full effect.

GOAL: Creating a cocoon, a peaceful resting state, but keeping your brain switched on. ← **READING/ JOURNALLING** → IDEA: Avoid vocals to keep attention on your task. Try classical music, or much slower ambient tracks.

GOAL: Time to move towards deeper rest, solitude, stillness and a quieter tone. ← **PRE-SLEEP** → IDEA: Use your ocean drum to evoke gentle waves before rest. Delta binaural beats are the win.

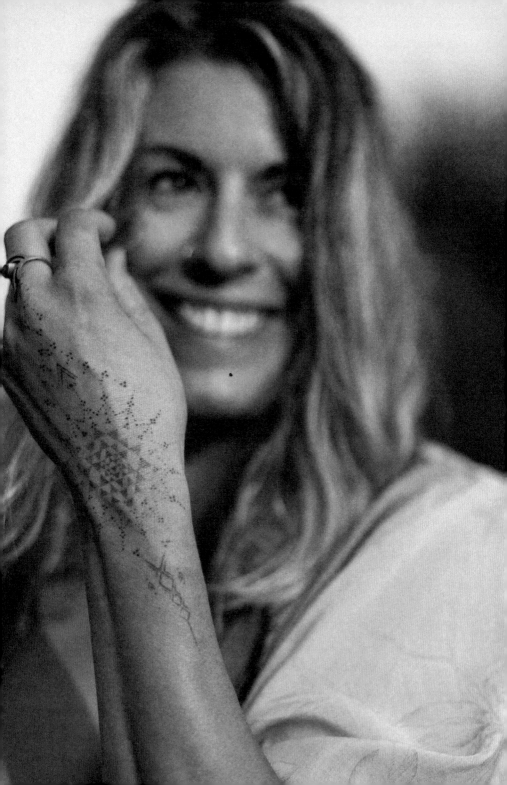

Your Sound Journey

" Sound is infused with intelligence, an organising principle that shapes the forms we perceive [even] through our eyes" Russill Paul, *The Yoga of Sound*

I hope that if this journey through the potency, power and potential of sound healing has left you with anything, it's the understanding that YOU are your own sound healer.

Whether you play an instrument, think you can't, want to learn, or don't think you ever will, really doesn't matter when it comes to sound.

Sound is simply presence, and you just have to be here now.

You can hear with your whole body, not just your ears.

And you can feel. Feel the physical impact of vibrations shimmering through your skin, and the emotional shifts as they ripple through your soul, reaching beyond consciousness.

From breathwork to fasting, plant medicine to sacred ceremony, humanity is gradually reconnecting with innate ancestral wisdom, and the healing power of sound sits at the very core of this eternal knowledge.

Alongside the return to nature's gifts, technology is enabling us to see, feel and experience the quantum field, supra-conscious states and the tangible impact of frequency like never before.

We may be 300,000 years or so into human evolution, but when it comes to sound healing, we're just getting started with the ultimate magic carpet ride.

Remember, the world is sound. Just like you.

SUPPLIERS & FURTHER READING

Recommended sound healing, sound therapy and energy work texts for further exploration:

Becoming Supernatural
Dr Joe Dispenza

Himalayan Sound Revelations
Frank Perry

In the Heart of the Gong Space
Sheila Whittaker

Sound Healing Farzana Ali

Sound Healing with Gongs Sheila Whittaker

Sound Medicine Kulreet Chaudhary

The Architecture of Sound
Jarrod Byrne Mayer

The Biology of Belief
Bruce Lipton

The Untethered Soul
Michael Singer

The World is Sound
Joachim Ernest Berendt

Tuning the Human Biofield
Eileen McKusick

Vibrational Medicine
Richard Gerber

The author recommends the following suppliers, some (but not all) of whom are featured in the photography for this book:

Adaptatrap Brighton
www.adaptatrap.co.uk

ADC Drums
www.adcdrums.co.uk

B Love Sacred Sound Flumies
www.blovesacredsound.co.uk

Dragonfly Percussion
www.dragonflypercussion.com

E-Cymbals
www.ecymbals.co.uk

Grotta Sonora Gongs
www.grottasonora.com

Koshi Chimes
www.koshi.fr/en/

Meinl Sonic Energy
www.meinlsonicenergy.com

Paiste Gongs
www.paistegongs.com

Tone of Life Gongs
www.toneoflifegongs.com

VERY SPECIAL THANKS
Himalayan Art Gallery Goa & Ladakh +91 85549 31061
(suppliers of directly sourced metal singing bowls and Himalayan crystal bowls, plus the gong featured in the book)
Laxmi Boutique @laxmi_boutique_goa

ACKNOWLEDGEMENTS
Thank you to my teachers over the years–especially Sheila, Phil and Bear. Thank you Lani for first introducing me to the gong, and Simone for showing me its potential; to Ali for inspiring me to play and to Leo for leading the way in modern sound healing.

Thank you to the thousands of people whose presence in my soundspaces has given me purpose, inspiration, invaluable feedback, direction and dharma.

Thank you London for being home, Cornwall for being the expansion, and India the destiny.

Thank you Madeleine for being my favourite tiny sound healer in training.

INDEX

A DAVID AND CHARLES BOOK
© David and Charles, Ltd 2024

David and Charles is an imprint of David and Charles, Ltd
Suite A, Tourism House, Pynes Hill, Exeter, EX2 5WS

Text and Designs © Janie Everett 2024
Layout and Illustration © David and Charles, Ltd 2024
Photography shot on location in Agonda, South Goa

First published in the UK and USA in 2024

A catalogue record for this book is available from the British Library.

ISBN-13: 9781446310601 paperback
ISBN-13: 9781446312193 EPUB

This book has been printed on paper from approved suppliers and made from
pulp from sustainable sources.

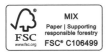

MIX
Paper | Supporting
responsible forestry
FSC
www.fsc.org   FSC® C106499

Printed in Turkey by Omur for:
David and Charles, Ltd, Suite A, Tourism House, Pynes Hill, Exeter, EX2 5WS

10 9 8 7 6 5 4 3 2 1

Publishing Director: Ame Verso
Senior Commissioning Editor: Lizzie Kaye
Managing Editor: Jeni Chown
Editor: Jessica Cropper
Project Editor: Jane Trollope
Head of Design: Anna Wade
Design and Illustration: Prudence Rogers
Photography: Mosalik Studios
Pre-press Designer: Susan Reansbury
Production Manager: Beverley Richardson

David and Charles publishes high-quality books on a wide range of subjects.
For more information visit www.davidandcharles.com.

Follow us on Instagram by searching for @dandcbooks_wellbeing.

Layout of the digital edition of this book may vary depending on reader
hardware and display settings.